GASTROPARESIS COOKBOOK

MEGA BUNDLE – 5 MANUSCRIPTS IN 1 – 240+ Gastroparesis-friendly recipes designed to manage Gastroparesis

TABLE OF CONTENTS

BREAKFAST 15
OMELET MUFFINS 15
BREAKFAST BURRITO 16
FRUIT AND YOGURT PARFAIT 17
STUFFED POTATO 18
COTTAGE CHEESE CUP 19
BREAKFAST SAUSAGE 20
BLUEBERRY PANCAKES 21
ALMOND POWDER PUDDING 22
BANANA COOKIES 23
EGG AND CHOCOLATE LOAF CAKE 24
EGG BENEDICT 26
STRAWBERRY SHORTCAKE 27
MORNING STRAWBERRY AND BERRIES PUREE 28
PEANUT BUTTER MILKSHAKE 29
GINGERBREAD PANCAKES 30
CINNAMON MUFFINS 31
MAPLE PUMPKIN BUTTER 33
PUMPKIN BUTTER TARTINE 34
ROASTED PEARS 35
JAMMY-FILLED MUFFINS 36
LUNCH 38
BUTTERMILK FRIED CHICKEN 38

ASIAN FISH EN PAPILLOTE	39
MAPLE GLAZED TURKEY BREAST	40
GARLIC MASHED POTATOES	41
STUFFING STOCK	42
MOIST ROAST CHICKEN	43
SPINACH FISH ROLLS	44
SPINACH PITA PIZZA	45
GAU'S CHICKEN	46
BUTTERNUT SQUASH STEW	47
SPINACH SALAD	49
TUNA SALAD	50
GREEN SALAD WITH THAI DRESSING	51
NOTATO SALAD	52
CUCUMBER SHRIMP SALAD	53
CITRUS FENNEL AND AVOCADO SALAD	54
STEAK SALAD	55
STEAK SALAD WITH ARUGULA	57
AVOCADO BACON SALAD	58
ASPARAGUS AND PROSCIUTTO SALAD	59
DINNER	60
ROASTED VEGETABLE PUREE	60
BANANA BREAD	61
HARDBOILED EGGS	62
WHIPPED SWEET POTATOES	63
BUTTERNUT SQUASH RISSOTTO	64
MAPLE GLAZED SWEET POTATOES	65

CARROT SOUFFLE 66

TANGY MASHED POTATOES 67

SHRIMP STOCK 68

OVEN ROASTED SCAMPI 69

SWEET POTATO SOUP 71

SWISS CHARD & SWEET POTATO SOUP 72

NO-COOK AVOCADO & MINT SOUP 73

HOMEMADE THAI CHICKEN BROTH 74

BLUEBERRY SOUP 75

ONION AND APPLE SOUP 76

CARROT SOUP 77

LIMA BEAN SOUP 78

ARTICHOKE AND LEEK SOUP 80

RICE SOUP 81

DESSERTS & SNACKS 82

PUMPKING CHOCOLATE CHIP COOKIES 82

CINNAMON TORTILLA CHIPS 84

BAKED BANANAS 85

NO-BAKE HOLLY TREATS 86

TARTAR BALLS 87

CHOCOLATE CHIP COOKIES 88

COCONUT MILK 90

ALMOND MILK 91

PROTEIN BAR 92

BANANA NOT CEREAL 93

CRANBERRY SMOOTHIE 94

CITRUS FLUSH	95
NO MILK SHAKE	96
CHERRY SHAKE	97
GOJI SMOOTHIE	98
ACAI SMOOTHIE	99
MATCHA TEA SMOOTHIE	100
PUMPKIN PIE SMOOTHIE	101
ALMOND SMOOTHIE	102
DECAF VANILLA TEA LATTE	103
GASTROPARESIS COOKBOOK	104
40+ Side Dishes, Salad and Pasta recipes designed for Gastroparesis	104
PASTA	105
LEMON PASTA	105
CHICKEN NOODLE SOUP	107
PASTA WITH NETTLE PESTO	109
CHICKEN PASTA	110
PASTA WITH BEEF	112
SATAY NOODLES	114
ZITI WITH MEAT SAUCE	116
NOODLE SOUP	118
SALAD	120
MORNING SALAD	120
COLESLAW	122
ASIAN BROCCOLI SALAD	123
GRILLED EGGPLANT AND FETA SALAD	124
SHRIMP AND AVOCADO SALAD	125

KALE SALAD WITH CITRUS-MAPLE VINAIGRETTE 126
GRILLED CORN SALAD 128
SIDE DISHES 129
AVOCADO TOAST 129
VEGGIE BURGERS 131
BROCCOLI SOUP 133
CRISPY DRUMSTICKS 134
BROILED SALMON 136
ROASTED ASPARAGUS 137
POTATO & CAULIFLOWER MASH 138
ROASTED BEETS 139
BAKED ZUCCHINI FRIES 140
CAULIFLOWER FRIED RICE 141
TABBOULEH 143
RED POTATOES & LEEKS 145
ROASTED CARROTS 146
OAT PORRIDGE 148
GUACAMOLE WITH PISTACHIOS 149
BAKED GREEN BEAN FRIES 150
COCONUT PINEAPPLE CASHEW RICE 151
GRILLED CORN 152
VEGETABLE KABOBS 153
SQUASH FRIES 155
ROASTED CAULIFLOWER 156
BANANA SNAPS 157
GINGER SOUP 159

ASIAN GREEN BEANS	161
ZUCCHINI WITH BALSAMIC REDUCTION	162
GASTROPARESIS COOKBOOK	165
40+ Smoothies, Dessert and Breakfast recipes designed for Gastroparesis	165
BREAKFAST	166
CHIA SEEDS WITH MAPLE SYRUP	166
COURGETTE SHAKSHUKA	167
MORNING SALAD	168
AVOCADO TOAST	169
GLUTEN-FREE BREAD	170
SAGE PATE	172
BANANA MUFFINS	173
KEDGEREE WITH TURMERIC	174
SUNFLOWER SEED PATE	176
WHITEBAIT FRITTERS	177
DESSERTS	178
PEARS POACHED WITH LEMON	178
BUTTER COOKIES	180
FROZEN STRAWBERRY CAKE	181
MANGO AND LIME SORBET	183
HONEY BAKED PLUMBS	184
PUMPKIN CARAMEL CAKE	186
LIME YOGURT CAKE	188
OAT PORRIDGE	190
ALMOND PANCAKES	191
BANANA SNAPS	192

SMOOTHIES 194

　BANANA BREAKFAST SMOOTHIE...194

　STRAWBERRY SUMMER SMOOTHIE 195

　RASPBERRY-ORANGE SMOOTHIE 196

　PEACH & MANGO SMOOTHIE 197

　CARROT MILKSHAKE 198

　CARROT SMOOTHIE 199

　CUCUMBER SMOOTHIE 200

　KIWI DETOX SMOOTHIE 201

　CHERRY SMOOTHIE..202

　MOCHA FAUXCCHINO...203

　ALMOND SMOOTHIE 204

　GRAPE SMOOTHIE 205

　PEAR SMOOTHIE...206

　GRAPEFRUIT SMOOTHIE...207

　PUMPKIN DETOX SMOOTHIE...208

　POMEGRANATE SMOOTHIE 209

　WATERMELON SMOOTHIE 210

　CELERY SMOOTHIE...211

　GINGER SMOOTHIE...212

　KIWI SMOOTHIE 2 213

GASTROPARESIS COOKBOOK...214

40+ Soup, pizza and side dishes recipes designed for Gastroparesis diet 214

SOUP RECIPES...215

　CABBAGE SOUP..215

　LENTIL SOUP 217

PUMPKIN SOUP 218

MUSHROOM SOUP 219

LEEK SOUP 221

BUTTERNUT SQUASH SOUP 222

OXTAIL SOUP 223

NOODLE SOUP 225

POTATO SOUP 227

BOLOGNESE SOUP WITH PENNE 229

CORIANDER SOUP 231

PASTA SOUP 232

CAULIFLOWER SOUP 234

BROCCOLI SOUP 236

CHEESE SOUP 238

LENTIL SOUP 239

WINTER SOUP 241

ROASTED RED PEPPER & SWEET POTATO SOUP 242

CELERY SOUP 244

TOMATO SOUP 245

PIZZA 247

GRAIN-FREE PIZZA CRUST 247

ZUCCHINI CRUST 249

BREAKFAST PIZZA 250

PIZZA WITH THE LOT 252

VEGGIE PIZZA WITH CAULIFLOWER CRUST 254

CAULIFLOWER PIZZA CRUST 256

COCONUT FLOUR PIZZA CRUST 258

PIZZA ROLLS	260
ZUCCHINI PIZZA CRUST	261
SPAGHETTI SQUASH PIZZA CRUST	263
LOW CARB ALMOND FLOUR PIZZA CRUST	264
SIDE DISHES	266
PAN SEARED SEA SCALLOPS	266
CHICKEN SAUTE	267
EGGS BENEDICT	269
GINGERBREAD SWEET POTATOES	270
HONEY ORANGE ROASTED BEETS	271
POPTART CRUMBLE	272
CRANBERRY GLAZED CHICKEN	273
ROASTED CHICKEN BREAST	275
KALE CHIPS	276
GARLIC HERB CRACKERS	277
GASTROPARESIS COOKBOOK	278
40+ Breakfast, pancakes, muffins and cookies recipes designed for Gastroparesis diet	278
BREAKFAST	279
CHIA SEEDS WITH MAPLE SYRUP	279
BAKED QUINOA WITH APPLES	280
FRIED HONEY BANANAS	281
PORTOBELLO EGGS	282
GLUTEN-FREE BREAD	284
BLUEBERRY JAM	286
ALMOND SMOOTHIE	287
CLASSIC FRIES	288

CHERRY KEFIR SMOOTHIE 290

CAULIFLOWER TORTILLAS 291

BROILED GRAPEFRUIT 292

BREAKFAST QUESADILLA 293

BAKED PEARS WITH WALNUTS 294

MOZZARELLA AND EGG BAKE 295

MORNING CARROT MILKSHAKE 296

BREAKFAST PEPPERS 297

AVOCADO BACON AND EGGS 299

APRICOT PROTEIN BAR 300

OAT PORRIDGE 301

COOKIES 302

BUTTER COOKIES 302

PANCAKES 304

ALMOND PANCAKES 304

OATMEAL PANCAKES 306

CLASSIC PANCAKES 308

FLUFFY PANCAKES 309

BUTTERMILK PANCAKES 310

RASPBERRY PANCAKES 311

BERRY PANCAKES 312

BANANA PANCAKES 313

VEGAN PANCAKES 314

OATMEAL-BANANA PANCAKES 315

MUFFINS 316

PUMPKIN PIE MUFFINS 316

5 MINUTE MUFFINS 318

BANANA MUFFINS 319

EGG MUFFINS 321

SIMPLE MUFFINS 323

BLUEBERRY MUFFINS 324

RASPBERRY MUFFINS 325

ALMOND MUFFINS 326

RAISIN MUFFINS 327

BACON MUFFINS 328

☐ Copyright 2019 by Noah Jerris - All rights reserved.

This document is geared towards providing exact and reliable information in regards to the topic and issue covered. The publication is sold with the idea that the publisher is not required to render accounting, officially permitted, or otherwise, qualified services. If advice is necessary, legal or professional, a practiced individual in the profession should be ordered.

- From a Declaration of Principles which was accepted and approved equally by a Committee of the American Bar Association and a Committee of Publishers and Associations.

In no way is it legal to reproduce, duplicate, or transmit any part of this document in either electronic means or in printed format. Recording of this publication is strictly prohibited and any storage of this document is not allowed unless with written permission from the publisher. All rights reserved.

The information provided herein is stated to be truthful and consistent, in that any liability, in terms of inattention or otherwise, by any usage or abuse of any policies, processes, or directions contained within is the solitary and utter responsibility of the recipient reader. Under no circumstances will any legal responsibility or blame be held against the publisher for any reparation, damages, or monetary loss due to the information herein, either directly or indirectly.

Respective authors own all copyrights not held by the publisher.

The information herein is offered for informational purposes solely, and is universal as so. The presentation of the information is without contract or any type of guarantee assurance.

The trademarks that are used are without any consent, and the publication of the trademark is without permission or backing by the trademark owner. All trademarks and brands within this book are for clarifying purposes only and are the owned by the owners themselves, not affiliated with this document.

Introduction

Gastroparesis recipes for personal enjoyment but also for family enjoyment. You will love them for sure for how easy it is to prepare them.

BREAKFAST

OMELET MUFFINS

Serves: *8*

Prep Time: *10* Minutes

Cook Time: *20* Minutes

Total Time: *30* Minutes

INGREDIENTS

- 2 eggs
- 5 egg whites
- 1 pinch of salt
- 1 tsp oregano
- 2 cups baby spinach

DIRECTIONS

1. Preheat the oven to 325 F
2. In a bowl mix eggs with egg whites, salt and pepper and oregano and copped baby spinach

3. Fill bottoms of muffin pans with baby spinach and fill with the eggs
4. Top with cheese and bake for 18-20 minutes
5. When ready, remove and serve

BREAKFAST BURRITO

Serves: 1
Prep Time: 5 Minutes
Cook Time: 5 Minutes
Total Time: 10 Minutes

INGREDIENTS

- 1 tablespoon salsa
- 1 tablespoon low-fat cheese
- 1 tortilla
- 1 scrambled egg

DIRECTIONS

1. Fill a tortilla with scrambled egg, cheese and salsa
2. Serve when ready

FRUIT AND YOGURT PARFAIT

Serves: 1

Prep Time: 5 Minutes

Cook Time: 5 Minutes

Total Time: 10 Minutes

INGREDIENTS

- ½ cup Greek yogurt
- ½ cup canned fruit
- ½ cup cherries

DIRECTIONS

1. **Top Greek yogurt with canned fruit**
2. **Add cherries and serve**

STUFFED POTATO

Serves: 2
Prep Time: **10** Minutes
Cook Time: **10** Minutes
Total Time: **20** Minutes

INGREDIENTS

- 1 baked potato
- 1 tablespoon chives
- 1 tablespoon tomatoes
- 1 tablespoon low-fat cheese
- 1 tablespoon Greek yogurt

DIRECTIONS

1. **Top a baked potato with a tomato, cheese, chives and Greek yogurt**
2. **Serve when ready**

COTTAGE CHEESE CUP

Serves: *1*

Prep Time: *5* Minutes

Cook Time: *5* Minutes

Total Time: *10* Minutes

INGREDIENTS

- ¾ cup low fat cottage cheese
- ¼ cup fruit canned
- ¼ cup sliced tomato

DIRECTIONS

1. In a bowl mix cottage cheese, ¼ cup fruit canned and also tomato slices
2. When ready, serve in the morning

BREAKFAST SAUSAGE

Serves: **6**

Prep Time: **10** Minutes

Cook Time: **20** Minutes

Total Time: **30** Minutes

INGREDIENTS

- 1 lb. turkey
- 1 tablespoon maple syrup
- 1 tsp salt
- ¾ tsp sage
- ¾ tsp thyme
- ½ tsp cinnamon

DIRECTIONS

1. Preheat the oven to 375 F
2. In a bowl mix all ingredients
3. Form 6-7 patties and place on a baking sheet
4. Bake for 15 minutes, remove and serve

BLUEBERRY PANCAKES

Serves: **4**

Prep Time: **10** Minutes

Cook Time: **10** Minutes

Total Time: **20** Minutes

INGREDIENTS

- 1 cup corn flour
- 1 tsp baking powder
- 1 cup plain yogurt
- 3 tablespoons coconut oil
- 2 eggs yolks
- 2 egg whites
- 1 tsp lemon zest
- 1 cup blueberries

DIRECTIONS

1. In a bowl mix dry ingredients and wet ingredients
2. In a skillet drop ¼ scoops of batter and add blueberries while cooking
3. Cook for 1-2 minutes or until golden brown
4. Remove and serve

ALMOND POWDER PUDDING

Serves: *3*

Prep Time: *10* Minutes

Cook Time: *10* Minutes

Total Time: *20* Minutes

INGREDIENTS

- ½ cup cottage cheese
- ½ cup fat free milk
- ¼ scoop chocolate protein powder
- ½ box chocolate instant pudding
- ½ tsp almond extract

DIRECTIONS

1. In a blender add cottage cheese and blend until smooth
2. Whisk remaining ingredients and blend until smooth
3. Divide into 2-3 servings and refrigerate
4. Garnish with cocoa powder and serve

BANANA COOKIES

Serves: **24**

Prep Time: **10** Minutes

Cook Time: **15** Minutes

Total Time: **25** Minutes

INGREDIENTS

- ½ cup butter
- 2 egg whites
- 1 tsp vanilla
- ¼ cup mashed banana
- ¼ cup brown sugar
- 1 cup flour
- 1 tsp baking powder
- ½ tsp salt
- ¼ tsp baking soda
- ¼ cup chocolate mini morsels

DIRECTIONS

1. Preheat the oven to 325 F
2. In a bowl mix butter, egg whites, mashed banana, vanilla, brown sugar and mix well

3. Add dry ingredients and mix well
4. Make small cookies and place on a baking sheet
5. Bake for 12-15 minutes or until golden brown
6. Remove cookies from the oven and serve

EGG AND CHOCOLATE LOAF CAKE

Serves: *8*
Prep Time: *10* Minutes

Cook Time: *35* Minutes

Total Time: *45* Minutes

INGREDIENTS

- **1 cup sugar**
- **1 cup flour**
- **¼ tsp salt**
- **½ cup cocoa powder**
- **1 tsp baking soda**
- **1 tablespoon white vinegar**
- **1 tablespoon canola oil**

- 1 container baby food prunes
- 1 tsp vanilla
- 1 cup boiling water

DIRECTIONS

1. Preheat the oven to 325 F
2. In a bowl sift together dry ingredients
3. In another bowl sift together wet ingredients and fold into dry ingredients
4. Pour mixture into a loaf pan and bake for 30-35 minutes, remove and serve

EGG BENEDICT

Serves: **2**

Prep Time: **10** Minutes

Cook Time: **10** Minutes

Total Time: **20** Minutes

INGREDIENTS
- 1 toaster waffle
- 1 triangle cow cheese
- chopped spinach
- 1 pinch salt
- 2 poached eggs

DIRECTIONS

1. Toast waffles and spread cow cheese
2. Top with poached eggs and spinach
3. Sprinkle salt and serve

STRAWBERRY SHORTCAKE

Serves: *1*

Prep Time: *10* Minutes

Cook Time: *10* Minutes

Total Time: *20* Minutes

INGREDIENTS

- 1 slice angel food cake
- 1 scoop strawberry sorbet
- 1 tablespoon fat free Reddi whip

DIRECTIONS

1. Preheat broiler
2. Toast angel food cake
3. Serve with a scoop of strawberry sorbet
4. Garnish with Reddi whip and serve

MORNING STRAWBERRY AND BERRIES PUREE

Serves: **4**
Prep Time: **10** Minutes
Cook Time: **30** Minutes
Total Time: **40** Minutes

INGREDIENTS

- 1 lb. strawberries
- 1 lb. berries

DIRECTIONS

1. **In a blender add strawberries and berries**
2. **Blend until smooth and serve**

PEANUT BUTTER MILKSHAKE

Serves: *1*
Prep Time: *5* Minutes
Cook Time: *5* Minutes
Total Time: *10* Minutes

INGREDIENTS

- ½ cup vanilla almond milk
- 1 tablespoon peanut butter
- 1 banana
- 1 oz. chocolate

DIRECTIONS

1. In a blender add all ingredients
2. Blend until smooth
3. Pour in a glass and serve

GINGERBREAD PANCAKES

Serves: **6**

Prep Time: **10** Minutes

Cook Time: **20** Minutes

Total Time: **30** Minutes

INGREDIENTS

- 1 tsp cinnamon
- ¾ tsp cloves
- 1 tsp ginger
- ½ tsp nutmeg
- 1 tablespoon molasses
- 1 tablespoon sugar
- 1 tsp vanilla
- zest of 1 lemon
- 1 tablespoon canola oil
- 1 egg
- 1 cup fat free milk

DIRECTIONS

1. In a bowl mix all ingredients

2. Pour ¼ cups batter onto a skillet
3. Cook for 1-2 minutes per side
4. Remove and serve

CINNAMON MUFFINS

Serves: **12**

Prep Time: **10** Minutes

Cook Time: **20** Minutes

Total Time: **30** Minutes

INGREDIENTS

- ¼ cup fat free sour cream
- 1 tablespoon lemon juice
- 1 tsp vanilla
- 1 tablespoon canola oil
- 2 egg whites
- 1 cup flour
- ¾ cups sugar
- 2 tsp baking powder

- ½ tsp salt
- 1 cup

STREUSEL TOPPING

- ½ cup brown sugar
- 1 tablespoon flour
- 1 tsp cinnamon
- 1 tablespoon butter

DIRECTIONS

1. Preheat the oven to 375 F and line a 12 cup muffin pan
2. In a bowl whisk dry ingredients and stir the wet ingredients into the dry, then stir well
3. Divide batter into the muffin cups
4. Pulse streusel ingredients until smooth and divide over each muffin
5. Bake for 15-20 minutes or until golden brown
6. Remove and serve

MAPLE PUMPKIN BUTTER

Serves: **1**

Prep Time: **10** Minutes

Cook Time: **20** Minutes

Total Time: **30** Minutes

INGREDIENTS

- 1 oz. can pumpkin puree
- ½ cup brown sugar
- 1 tablespoon maple syrup
- ½ cup water
- ¼ tsp cinnamon
- ½ tsp ginger
- ½ tsp nutmeg

DIRECTIONS

1. In a saucepan add all ingredients and bring to a boil
2. Cook over medium heat for 15-18 minutes
3. Remove from heat and pour into a jar
4. Refrigerate for 3-4 hours before serving

PUMPKIN BUTTER TARTINE

Serves: 2
Prep Time: 10 Minutes
Cook Time: 10 Minutes
Total Time: 20 Minutes

INGREDIENTS

- 1 low fat toaster wafer
- maple pumpkin butter
- ½ cup cottage cheese
- canned peach slices

DIRECTIONS

1. **Toast waffle**
2. **Spread maple pumpkin butter**
3. **Top with cottage cheese and sliced peaches**
4. **Serve when ready**

ROASTED PEARS

Serves: 2
Prep Time: 10 Minutes
Cook Time: 45 Minutes
Total Time: 55 Minutes

INGREDIENTS

- 2 pears
- juice of ½ lemon
- 1 pinch of salt

DIRECTIONS

1. Preheat the oven to 375 F
2. Toss pears in lemon juice
3. Season with salt and pepper and roast for 40-45 minutes
4. Remove to a cutting board, cut into slices and serve

JAMMY-FILLED MUFFINS

Serves: **12**

Prep Time: **10** Minutes

Cook Time: **20** Minutes

Total Time: **30** Minutes

INGREDIENTS

- 1 cup flour
- ¼ cup sugar
- ¼ tsp salt
- 1 tablespoon baking powder
- 1 cup fat free milk
- 1 tsp vanilla
- zest of 1 lemon
- 1 egg
- 5 tablespoons raspberry jam

DIRECTIONS

1. Preheat the oven to 475 F and line a 12 cup muffin pan
2. In a bowl mix dry ingredients and fold in wet ingredients and lemon zest
3. Mix well and fill muffin cups with 1/3 batter

4. Fill 1/3 with jam and bake for 18-20 minutes or until golden brown
5. When ready, remove from the oven and serve

LUNCH

BUTTERMILK FRIED CHICKEN

Serves: *4*

Prep Time: *10* Minutes

Cook Time: *20* Minutes

Total Time: *30* Minutes

INGREDIENTS

- 2 chicken breasts
- ½ cup low fat buttermilk
- salt free seasoning
- ¼ cup bread crumbs
- salt

DIRECTIONS

1. Preheat the oven to 400 F
2. Cut chicken breast in half and marinate in buttermilk and seasoning for 45-60 minutes
3. Dredge each piece of chicken in crumbs and coat well
4. Place chicken on a sheet pan and bake for 12-15 minutes or until golden
5. When ready, remove and serve

ASIAN FISH EN PAPILLOTE

Serves: 1
Prep Time: 10 Minutes
Cook Time: 20 Minutes
Total Time: 30 Minutes

INGREDIENTS

- 2 tsp soy sauce
- 2 tsp rice wine vinegar
- 1 tablespoon ginger root
- 5 oz. fillet white fish
- 2 green onions

DIRECTIONS

1. Preheat the oven to 400 F
2. In a bowl mix ginger, rice wine vinegar and soy sauce
3. Place the fish fillet on the parchment paper and top with green onion and drizzle with soy mixture
4. Top with mushrooms, jasmine rice and bake for 10-15 minutes, when ready, remove and serve

MAPLE GLAZED TURKEY BREAST

Serves: **6**

Prep Time: **10** Minutes

Cook Time: **1** Hour 30 Minutes

Total Time: **1** Hour 40 Minutes

INGREDIENTS

- 5 lbs. turkey breast
- 1 recipe wild mushrooms
- 1 tablespoon maple syrup

DIRECTIONS

1. Preheat the oven to 375 F
2. Place the turkey breast on a butting board and season with salt and pepper
3. Place stuffing in the center of the pan
4. Roast for 1 hour and 30 minutes
5. Remove, brush with maple syrup and allow to rest before serving

GARLIC MASHED POTATOES

Serves: **4**

Prep Time: **10** Minutes

Cook Time: **30** Minutes

Total Time: **40** Minutes

INGREDIENTS

- 6 potatoes
- ½ cup milk
- ½ cup butter
- 1 clove garlic
- 1 pinch of salt
- 1 pinch ground black pepper
- 1 tablespoon sesame seeds

DIRECTIONS

1. In a pot bring water to boil, add potatoes and boil for 25 minutes
2. In a bowl mix pepper, garlic, milk, butter and salt with a hand mixer
3. Sprinkle with sesame seeds and serve with mashed potatoes

STUFFING STOCK

Serves: **6**

Prep Time: **10** Minutes

Cook Time: **2** Hours

Total Time: **2** Hours 10 Minutes

INGREDIENTS

- 6 cups chicken stock
- 2 onions
- 2 stalks celery
- spring parsley
- 1 bay leaf
- 4 peppercorns
- mushroom steams

DIRECTIONS

1. In a pot add all ingredients and cover with a lid
2. Bring mixture to a boil and simmer for 2 hours
3. When ready remove from heat
4. Refrigerate and serve

MOIST ROAST CHICKEN

Serves: **4**

Prep Time: **10** Minutes

Cook Time: **30** Minutes

Total Time: **40** Minutes

INGREDIENTS

- 2 chicken breasts
- salt
- pepper

DIRECTIONS

1. Preheat the oven to 400 F
2. Place chicken breast on a cutting board and season with salt and pepper
3. Roast for 30 minutes
4. Remove and serve when ready

SPINACH FISH ROLLS

Serves: **4**

Prep Time: **10** Minutes

Cook Time: **20** Minutes

Total Time: **30** Minutes

INGREDIENTS

- 1 lb. fillets
- seasoning
- 1 cup spinach
- 1 cup mayonnaise
- plain bread crumbs
- 1 tablespoon white vermouth

DIRECTIONS

1. Preheat the oven to 375 F
2. Season fish fillets with seasoning and chopped spinach
3. Roll fillets and top each roll with mayonnaise and a sprinkle of bread crumbs
4. Add vermouth to the baking dish and bake for 18-20 minutes, remove and serve with lemon wedges

SPINACH PITA PIZZA

Serves: 4
Prep Time: 10 Minutes
Cook Time: 20 Minutes
Total Time: 30 Minutes

INGREDIENTS

- 1 white pizza
- strained pizza sauce
- 1 tablespoon Italian seasoning
- 1 tablespoon spinach
- ½ cup cottage cheese
- 1 oz. mozzarella cheese

DIRECTIONS

1. Preheat the oven to 375 F
2. Toast pita and spread tomato space over
3. Sprinkle with seasoning, spinach, mozzarella and cottage cheese
4. Return to oven and bake until cheese is fully melted
5. When ready, remove from oven and serve

GAU'S CHICKEN

Serves: **4**

Prep Time: **10** Minutes

Cook Time: **20** Minutes

Total Time: **30** Minutes

INGREDIENTS

- 1 tablespoon cornstarch
- ¼ cup water
- 2 garlic cloves
- 2 tsp ginger root
- 2 tablespoons brown sugar
- 2 tablespoons soy sauce
- 1 tablespoon orange juice
- 1 lb. chicken breast

DIRECTIONS

1. In a bowl mix all ingredients except chicken breast
2. Season chicken breast with salt and pepper
3. Sauté chicken in large wok for 2-3 minutes
4. Add cornstarch mixture and cook for another 5-6 minutes

5. When ready, remove from heat and serve

BUTTERNUT SQUASH STEW

Serves: **4**

Prep Time: **10** Minutes

Cook Time: **30** Minutes

Total Time: **40** Minutes

INGREDIENTS

- 2 tsp olive oil
- 1 clove garlic
- 2 cups butternut squash
- 1 cup carrots
- 2 cups chicken broth
- ¼ tsp thyme
- 1 bay leaf
- ½ tsp salt
- 8 oz. chicken breast
- ¼ tsp onion powder

- 1 pinch nutmeg
- 1 tablespoon orange juice concentrate

DIRECTIONS

1. In a Dutch oven add garlic, olive oil, carrots, squash cubes and cook for 4-5 minutes
2. Stir in thyme, salt, bay leaf, broth and bring to a boil
3. Simmer for 15-20 minutes, until vegetables are tender
4. Remove 1 cup and puree, return to the pan and bring to a boil
5. Add chicken cubes, orange juice, nutmeg and simmer for another 5-6 minutes
6. When ready, remove from heat and serve

SPINACH SALAD

Serves: **2**
Prep Time: **5** Minutes
Cook Time: **5** Minutes
Total Time: **10** Minutes

INGREDIENTS

- 2 oranges
- 1 grapefruit
- 5 cups baby spinach
- 3 scallions 3 oz. prosciutto

DRESSING

- 2 tablespoons balsamic vinegar
- 2 tablespoons olive oil
- 2 tablespoons cream
- 2 tsp honey
- ½ tsp salt
- ½ tsp black pepper

DIRECTIONS

1. In a bowl mix all ingredients and mix well
2. Serve with dressing

TUNA SALAD

Serves: 2
Prep Time: 5 Minutes
Cook Time: 5 Minutes
Total Time: 10 Minutes

INGREDIENTS

- 2 cups cooked pasta
- ½ cup celery
- 2 tablespoons bell pepper
- 2 tablespoons green onion
- 1 tsp lemon zest
- ½ cup low fat mayonnaise
- ½ cup Italian salad dressing
- 4 oz. canned tuna

DIRECTIONS

1. In a bowl mix all ingredients and mix well
2. Serve with dressing

GREEN SALAD WITH THAI DRESSING

Serves: 2
Prep Time: 5 Minutes
Cook Time: 5 Minutes
Total Time: 10 Minutes

INGREDIENTS

- 2 cucumber
- 10 cups salad greens
- 2 cups sunflower sprouts
- 2 stalks celery

DRESSING

- ½ cup lime juice
- 2 tablespoons fish sauce
- ¼ tsp honey
- 1 clove garlic
- 1 tablespoon cilantro

DIRECTIONS

1. In a bowl mix all ingredients and mix well
2. Serve with dressing

NOTATO SALAD

Serves: **4**

Prep Time: **10** Minutes

Cook Time: **30** Minutes

Total Time: **40** Minutes

INGREDIENTS

- 3 cups turnip
- 3 cups sweet potato
- 3cup stalks celery
- ½ cup red onion

DRESSING

- 2 tablespoons palm shortening
- 1 tsp salt
- ½ tsp turmeric
- ½ tsp wasabi powder
- 2 tablespoons olive oil
- 1 tsp dried dill
- 1 tablespoon lemon juice

DIRECTIONS

1. In a bowl mix all ingredients and mix well
2. Serve with dressing

CUCUMBER SHRIMP SALAD

Serves: 2
Prep Time: 5 Minutes
Cook Time: 5 Minutes
Total Time: 10 Minutes

INGREDIENTS

- 1 lb. shrimp
- 1 cucumber
- ½ cup red onion
- ½ cup mango
- ¼ cup cilantro

DRESSING

- ½ cup olive oil
- ½ cup lime juice

- 1 tablespoon honey
- 1 clove garlic
- 1 tsp salt

DIRECTIONS

1. In a bowl mix all ingredients and mix well
2. Serve with dressing

CITRUS FENNEL AND AVOCADO SALAD

Serves: 2
Prep Time: 5 Minutes
Cook Time: 5 Minutes
Total Time: 10 Minutes

INGREDIENTS

- 5 cups baby greens
- 1 bulb fennel
- ¼ cup red onion

- 1 orange
- 1 grapefruit
- 6 cooked salmon fillet
- ¼ avocado
- ½ tsp garlic granules

DIRECTIONS

1. In a bowl mix all ingredients and mix well
2. Serve with dressing

STEAK SALAD

Serves: 2
Prep Time: 5 Minutes
Cook Time: 5 Minutes
Total Time: 10 Minutes

INGREDIENTS

- 1 lb. grassfed steaks

- 1 tablespoon coconut oil
- 3 handful greens
- 3 oz. mushrooms
- 1 handful Italian parsley

DRESSING
- ¼ cup olive oil
- 2 tablespoons balsamic vinegar
- 2 tablespoons tarragon
- ½ tsp garlic powder
- ¼ tsp salt

DIRECTIONS

1. In a bowl mix all ingredients and mix well
2. Serve with dressing

STEAK SALAD WITH ARUGULA

Serves: 2
Prep Time: 5 Minutes
Cook Time: 5 Minutes
Total Time: 10 Minutes

INGREDIENTS

- 10 oz. steak
- 4 oz. baby arugula
- juice of 1 lemon
- 1 tablespoon olive oil
- 1 tsp salt

DIRECTIONS

1. In a bowl mix all ingredients and mix well
2. Serve with dressing

AVOCADO BACON SALAD

Serves: 2

Prep Time: 5 Minutes

Cook Time: 5 Minutes

Total Time: 10 Minutes

INGREDIENTS

- 1 head broccoli
- 2 stalks celery
- 3 slices bacon
- ½ cup red onion
- 1 tablespoon raisins
- 1 avocado
- 1 tablespoon apple cider vinegar
- 1 tsp salt
- 1 tsp black pepper

DIRECTIONS

1. In a bowl mix all ingredients and mix well
2. Serve with dressing

ASPARAGUS AND PROSCIUTTO SALAD

Serves: 2

Prep Time: 5 Minutes

Cook Time: 5 Minutes

Total Time: 10 Minutes

INGREDIENTS

- 2 chicken breasts
- 2 tsp olive oil
- 3 slices prosciutto
- 5 asparagus spears
- 1 handful arugula leaves
- 1 avocado
- 1 tablespoon olive oil
- 1 garlic clove
- juice of 1 lime

DIRECTIONS

1. In a bowl mix all ingredients and mix well
2. Serve with dressing

DINNER

ROASTED VEGETABLE PUREE

Serves: **4**

Prep Time: **10** Minutes

Cook Time: **50** Minutes

Total Time: **60** Minutes

INGREDIENTS

- 2 lbs. sweet potatoes
- 1 lb. white potatoes
- ¼ lb. carrots
- 1 tablespoon olive oil
- 1,5 cup vegetable stock

DIRECTIONS

1. Preheat the oven to 350 F
2. Toss vegetables with olive oil and place in a roasting pan
3. Pour 1 cup of broth and roast for 45-50 minutes or until tender
4. Remove and puree vegetables with remaining broth and serve

BANANA BREAD

Serves: *12*

Prep Time: *10* Minutes

Cook Time: *40* Minutes

Total Time: *50* Minutes

INGREDIENTS

- 2 bananas
- ¾ cup pure maple syrup
- ½ cup coconut oil
- 1 tsp pure vanilla extract
- 1 cup flour
- ½ cup cocoa powder
- 1 tsp baking soda
- ½ tsp salt

DIRECTIONS

1. Preheat the oven to 325 F
2. In a bowl add mashed bananas, coconut oil, vanilla extract and maple syrup and mix well
3. In a bowl mix salt, flour, cocoa, baking soda and add to banana mixture and mix well

4. Pour batter into pan and bake for 40 minutes
5. When ready, remove and serve

HARDBOILED EGGS

Serves: **4**

Prep Time: **10** Minutes

Cook Time: **30** Minutes

Total Time: **40** Minutes

INGREDIENTS

- 4 eggs

DIRECTIONS

1. Preheat the oven to 300 F
2. In a muffin pan place 4 eggs and cook for 25-30 minutes
3. When eggs are done, transfer to a bowl of cold water, allow to cool, peel and store

WHIPPED SWEET POTATOES

Serves: 6

Prep Time: 10 Minutes

Cook Time: 60 Minutes

Total Time: 70 Minutes

INGREDIENTS

- 2 lbs. sweet potatoes
- ½ cup orange juice
- ¼ cup water
- 1 tablespoon coconut oil
- 1 tsp cinnamon
- 1 tsp salt

DIRECTIONS

1. Preheat the oven to 350 F
2. Place sweet potatoes on a baking sheet
3. Bake for 50-60 minutes, remove and slice each potato in half
4. Add all ingredients in a blender, blend until smooth and serve

BUTTERNUT SQUASH RISSOTTO

Serves: **4**

Prep Time: **10** Minutes

Cook Time: **20** Minutes

Total Time: **30** Minutes

INGREDIENTS

- 1 cup uncooked rice
- 1 tsp olive oil
- 2 cups chicken broth
- 1 cup butternut squash
- 1 pinch of salt
- 1 pinch of black pepper
- 5 tablespoons Parmesan cheese

DIRECTIONS

1. In a bowl mix rice, oil and microwave for 3-4 minutes
2. Add broth, water and microwave for 8-10 minutes
3. Add salt, pepper, squash, cheese risotto and stir well
4. Serve when ready

MAPLE GLAZED SWEET POTATOES

Serves: **8**

Prep Time: **10** Minutes

Cook Time: **60** Minutes

Total Time: **70** Minutes

INGREDIENTS

- 2 lbs. sweet potatoes
- ¼ tsp salt
- ½ cup maple syrup

DIRECTIONS

1. Preheat the oven to 325 F
2. Sprinkle potato slices with salt and arrange in the baking dish
3. Pour maple syrup over the potatoes
4. Bake for 60 minutes or until golden brown
5. Remove and serve

CARROT SOUFFLE

Serves: **8**

Prep Time: **10** Minutes

Cook Time: **55** Minutes

Total Time: **65** Minutes

INGREDIENTS

- 2 lbs. baby carrots
- 2/3 cups granulated sugar
- ½ cup sour cream
- 2 tablespoons flour
- 1 tablespoon butter
- 1 tsp baking powder
- 1 tsp vanilla extract
- ½ tsp salt
- ¾ cup egg beaters

DIRECTIONS

1. Preheat the oven to 25 F
2. Slice the carrots and bake for 12-15 minutes or until tender
3. Place carrots in a blender and blend until smooth

4. Add all ingredients except salt and egg beaters and blend again
5. Spoon mixture into a baking dish and bake for another 40 minutes
6. Remove and serve

TANGY MASHED POTATOES

Serves: *4*
Prep Time: *10* Minutes
Cook Time: *20* Minutes
Total Time: *30* Minutes

INGREDIENTS

- 2 lb. gold potatoes
- 5 oz. chicken broth
- 5 oz. low-fat Greek Yogurt
- 1 tsp salt

DIRECTIONS

1. Boil potatoes until tender
2. Mash potatoes, add broth, sour cream and mix well, season and serve when ready

SHRIMP STOCK

Serves: 2

Prep Time: **10** Minutes

Cook Time: **30** Minutes

Total Time: **40** Minutes

INGREDIENTS

- 2 cups water
- 2 lbs. raw shrimp
- 2 bay leaves
- ½ lemon
- 1 onion
- 1 clove garlic
- 1 fresh thyme
- 1 fresh tarragon

- 1 pinch red pepper flakes

DIRECTIONS

1. In a saucepan place all ingredients and bring to a boil
2. Simmer for 25-30 minutes
3. Strain and cool
4. Serve when ready

OVEN ROASTED SCAMPI

Serves: *4*
Prep Time: *10* Minutes

Cook Time: *30* Minutes

Total Time: *40* Minutes

INGREDIENTS

- 2 lbs. shrimp
- 2 cloves garlic
- 1 tablespoon butter

- springs of thyme
- 1 cup shrimp stock
- ½ cup dry vermouth
- 1 tablespoon lemon juice
- zest of 1 lemon
- 1 pinch of salt

DIRECTIONS

1. Preheat the oven to 450 F
2. In a bowl mix garlic, butter and set aside
3. In a baking dish place the shrimp and springs of thyme over shrimp
4. In a bowl mix lemon zest, lemon juice, shrimp stock, vermouth and season with pepper and salt and pour over shrimp
5. Place garlic mixture over shrimp
6. Bake until tender
7. Toss to coat shrimp with sauce and serve

SWEET POTATO SOUP

Serves: **4**

Prep Time: **10** Minutes

Cook Time: **30** Minutes

Total Time: **40** Minutes

INGREDIENTS

- 2 sweet potatoes
- 3 cups vegetable broth
- ¼ cup onion
- 1 cup kale
- 1 tsp paprika
- 1 tsp garlic powder
- ¼ tsp ginger
- 1 tablespoon olive oil
- 1 tsp salt

DIRECTIONS

1. Preheat the oven to 350 F
2. Microwave sweet potatoes for 10-12 minutes, then bake for 20 minutes
3. Remove from the oven and place them in a blender

4. Add the rest of ingredients and blend until smooth
5. Transfer soup to a soup pot and cook on low heat
6. Add kale leaves and simmer until ready to serve

SWISS CHARD & SWEET POTATO SOUP

Serves: **4**

Prep Time: **10** Minutes

Cook Time: **30** Minutes

Total Time: **40** Minutes

INGREDIENTS

- 1 cup duck fat
- 1 onion
- 1,5 lbs. zucchini
- 1 oz. sweet potato
- 3 cups bone broth
- 1 Swiss chard
- 1 bunch cilantro
- ½ lemon juice

DIRECTIONS

1. In a saucepan add onions and sauté for 10 minutes
2. Add sweet potato, zucchini and stir to coat
3. Add bone broth and the rest of ingredients and cook on low heat until potato is soft
4. Pure soup until smooth
5. Return soup to the saucepan and cook until ready to serve

NO-COOK AVOCADO & MINT SOUP

Serves: *4*
Prep Time: *10* Minutes
Cook Time: *10* Minutes
Total Time: *20* Minutes

INGREDIENTS

- 1 avocado
- 2 romaine lettuce leaves
- 1 cup coconut milk

- 1 tablespoon lime juice
- 16-18 mint leaves
- salt

DIRECTIONS

1. Place all ingredients in a blender and blend until smooth
2. Pour in a bowl and place in the fridge for 10-15 before serving

HOMEMADE THAI CHICKEN BROTH

Serves: *8*
Prep Time: *10* Minutes

Cook Time: *10* Minutes

Total Time: *20* Minutes

INGREDIENTS

- 1 chicken
- 1 stalk lemongrass

- 16-18 basil leaves
- 4 slices ginger
- 1 lime
- 1 tsp salt

DIRECTIONS

1. In a slow cooker add chicken, lemon grass, basil leaves and cook on low for 8-10 hours
2. Ladle the broth into a bowl, add salt, lime juice and garnish basil leaves
3. Serve when ready

BLUEBERRY SOUP

Serves: *4*
Prep Time: *10* Minutes
Cook Time: *60* Minutes
Total Time: *70* Minutes

INGREDIENTS

- 2 cups blueberries
- 1 can coconut milk
- ¼ tsp rosemary
- ½ tsp cinnamon
- 1 tablespoon apple cider vinegar
- 1 tablespoon lemon juice
- 1 pinch salt

DIRECTIONS

1. In a pot add all ingredients and cook for 10-12 minutes
2. Allow to cook for 30 minutes
3. Pour soup in a blender and blend until smooth
4. Pour in a bowl and garnish with rosemary

ONION AND APPLE SOUP

Serves: **4**

Prep Time: **10** Minutes

Cook Time: **30** Minutes

Total Time: **40** Minutes

INGREDIENTS

- 1 tablespoon canola oil
- 1 onion
- 1 leek
- ¼ tablespoon rosemary
- ¼ tablespoon thyme
- 2 apples
- 5 cup vegetable broth

DIRECTIONS

1. In a saucepan heat oil over medium heat, add onions and sauté for 4-5 minutes
2. Pour in the broth and bring to boil, add apples and reduce heat
3. Simmer until soup is ready, remove from heat and serve

CARROT SOUP

Serves: **4**

Prep Time: **10** Minutes

Cook Time: **30** Minutes

Total Time: **40** Minutes

INGREDIENTS

- 2 beets
- 1 tablespoon olive oil
- 1 onion
- 1 lb. carrots
- 1 tablespoon ginger
- 1 garlic clove
- 5 cups vegetable broth

DIRECTIONS

1. In a saucepan sauté onion until golden brown
2. Add ginger, garlic and cook for 2-3 minutes
3. Add beets, carrots and stock and simmer on low heat for 25-30 minutes
4. Puree soup in batches
5. Remove, garnish with cilantro leaves and serve

LIMA BEAN SOUP

Serves: **4**
Prep Time: **10** Minutes
Cook Time: **30** Minutes
Total Time: **40** Minutes

INGREDIENTS

- 10 oz. lima beans
- 1 tablespoon butter
- 1 bunch scallion
- 1 tsp curry powder
- 1 tsp salt
- ¼ tsp pepper
- ¼ tsp dried tarragon
- 3 springs parsley
- 2 cups chicken broth
- ¼ cup skim milk

DIRECTIONS

1. In a blender add butter, scallions, lima beans, curry powder, tarragon, parsley, salt and blend until smooth
2. Place mixture into a pot, add milk, broth and simmer for 12-15 minutes
3. Pour soup into bowls and serve

ARTICHOKE AND LEEK SOUP

Serves: **4**

Prep Time: **10** Minutes

Cook Time: **30** Minutes

Total Time: **40** Minutes

INGREDIENTS

- 12 oz. artichoke hearts
- 1 cup sliced leeks
- 2 cups chicken broth
- 2 tablespoons sour cream

DIRECTIONS

1. In a blender add artichoke hearts and blend until smooth
2. In a pot add leeks, artichoke hearts and cook for 10-12 minutes
3. Add chicken broth and simmer for 12-15 minutes on medium heat

4. Place soup into a blender and blend until smooth
5. Pour into bowls and serve with sour cream

RICE SOUP

Serves: **4**

Prep Time: **10** Minutes

Cook Time: **30** Minutes

Total Time: **40** Minutes

INGREDIENTS

- 1 cup onion
- 1 cup celery
- 1 cup baby carrot
- 1 tablespoon olive oil
- 1/3 cup white rice
- black pepper
- 3 thyme springs
- 1 bay leaf
- 10 cups no-salt chicken broth

- 2 cooked chicken breats
- 2 tablespoons lime juice

DIRECTIONS

1. In a soup pot add all soup ingredients
2. Sauté for 5-6 minutes
3. Add water simmer for 20-30 minutes
4. Season with pepper
5. When ready, pour into bowls and serve

DESSERTS & SNACKS

PUMPKING CHOCOLATE CHIP COOKIES

Serves: **20**
Prep Time: **10** Minutes

Cook Time: **20** Minutes

Total Time: **30** Minutes

INGREDIENTS

- 1 box vanilla cake mix
- 1 can sweet potato puree
- 1 tsp cinnamon
- ¼ tsp ginger
- 1 tsp cinnamon
- ½ tsp vanilla extract
- ¼ cup cacao chocolate chips

DIRECTIONS

1. Preheat the oven to 325 F
2. In a bowl mix spices, cake mix, puree and vanilla
3. Stir in chocolate chips and drop onto a cookie sheet
4. Bake for 8-10 minutes, remove and set aside
5. Puree sweet potato and mix with the rest ingredients
6. Bake for another 8-10 minutes
7. Remove and serve

CINNAMON TORTILLA CHIPS

Serves: **4**

Prep Time: **10** Minutes

Cook Time: **30** Minutes

Total Time: **40** Minutes

INGREDIENTS

- 8 flour tortillas
- 1 tablespoon water
- ½ cup sugar
- 2 tsp cinnamon

DIRECTIONS

1. Preheat the oven to 375 F
2. In a bowl mix sugar and cinnamon
3. Brush tortillas with water and sprinkle with cinnamon mixture
4. Cut each tortilla into 6-8 wedges
5. Bake for 8-10 minutes, remove and serve

BAKED BANANAS

Serves: **4**

Prep Time: **5** Minutes

Cook Time: **15** Minutes

Total Time: **20** Minutes

INGREDIENTS

- 3 bananas
- 1 tsp coconut oil
- 1-inch fresh ginger
- 1 tablespoon cinnamon
- ¼ tablespoon nutmeg
- 3 tablespoon sugar

DIRECTIONS

1. **Preheat the oven to 350 F**
2. **Cut bananas in half lengthwise**
3. **In a baking pan arrange bananas and sprinkle with cinnamon, ginger, nutmeg and sugar**
4. **Bake for 12-15 minutes, remove and serve**

NO-BAKE HOLLY TREATS

Serves: **6**

Prep Time: **10** Minutes

Cook Time: **55** Minutes

Total Time: **65** Minutes

INGREDIENTS

- 2 tablespoons butter
- 20-30 marshmallows
- 1 tsp vanilla
- food coloring
- 3 cups corn flakes
- red hot cinnamon candies

DIRECTIONS

1. In a pot melt butter, marshmallow and stir in vanilla, food coloring and mix well

2. In a bowl beat butter, sugar, egg whites, maple syrup and vanilla and blend
3. Add corn flakes, and drop bunches onto waxed paper, allow to chill for 50-60 minutes before serving

TARTAR BALLS

Serves: **4**

Prep Time: **10** Minutes

Cook Time: **30** Minutes

Total Time: **40** Minutes

INGREDIENTS

- **1 cup all-purpose flour**
- **¼ tsp baking soda**
- **¼ tsp cream of tartar**
- **¾ cup sugar**
- **½ cup butter**
- **½ cup pure maple syrup**
- **1 tsp vanilla**

- ½ cup egg whites
- 2 tablespoons sugar
- 2 tsp cinnamon

DIRECTIONS

1. Preheat the oven to 350 F
2. In a bowl mix baking soda, flour and cream of tartar
3. In a bowl add maple syrup, sugar, egg whites and vanilla
4. Add flour mixture to sugar mixture and mix well
5. Form dough into balls and roll each ball in cinnamon
6. Place balls on a baking sheet and bake for 8-10 minutes
7. Remove and serve

CHOCOLATE CHIP COOKIES

Serves: **4**
Prep Time: **10** Minutes
Cook Time: **30** Minutes

Total Time: *40* Minutes

INGREDIENTS

- 2 cups gluten free oats
- ¼ cup palm oil
- ½ cup coconut oil
- ½ cup maple syrup
- ½ cup sucanat
- 1 tsp vanilla extract
- 1 tsp baking powder
- ½ cup cup chocolate chips

DIRECTIONS

1. Preheat the oven to 350 F
2. Place oats in a blender and blend until they become flour
3. In a bowl mix vanilla, sucanat, maple syrup, cream oils and fold in chocolate chips
4. Scoop mixture onto the baking sheet and bake for 10-12 minutes
5. Remove and serve

COCONUT MILK

Serves: **1**
Prep Time: **5** Minutes
Cook Time: **5** Minutes
Total Time: **10** Minutes

INGREDIENTS

- 2 cups unsweetened milk
- 5 cups water
- 1 cup coconut flakes

DIRECTIONS

1. Soak coconut flakes for 1-2 hours
2. Pour coconut flakes and unsweetened milk into your blender
3. Add water and blend until smooth
4. Pour into a jar and refrigerate

ALMOND MILK

Serves: *1*

Prep Time: *5* Minutes

Cook Time: *1* Minutes

Total Time: *10* Minutes

INGREDIENTS

- 1 cup almonds
- 8 cups water
- 1 pinch salt
- 1 tsp vanilla extract
- maple syrup

DIRECTIONS

1. In a bowl add water, almonds and soak overnight
2. Drain and rise almonds and place in a blender
3. Add sweetener, salt, and blend until smooth
4. Pour into a jar and refrigerate

PROTEIN BAR

Serves: 6
Prep Time: 10 Minutes
Cook Time: 25 Minutes
Total Time: 35 Minutes

INGREDIENTS

- 1 cup quinoa flakes
- ¼ cup sunflower seed butter
- 1 scoop unsweetened protein powder
- ½ cup maple syrup
- 2 tablespoons coconut milk

DIRECTIONS

1. **In a bowl mix maple syrup, sunflower seed butter, protein powder, quinoa flakes and mix well**
2. **Add coconut milk and spread onto a loaf pan**
3. **Bake for 20-25 minutes**
4. **When ready, remove and slice into 6-8 bars**

BANANA NOT CEREAL

Serves: *4*
Prep Time: *10* Minutes
Cook Time: *30* Minutes
Total Time: *40* Minutes

INGREDIENTS

- ½ cup hot cereal
- 1 cup water
- ¼ mashed banana
- 1 tablespoon hazelnut butter
- cinnamon

DIRECTIONS

1. In a saucepan boil water, add cereal and simmer for 10-15 minutes
2. Remove from heat stir in hazelnut butter, cinnamon and bananas
3. Serve when ready

CRANBERRY SMOOTHIE

Serves: 1
Prep Time: 5 Minutes
Cook Time: 5 Minutes
Total Time: 10 Minutes

INGREDIENTS

- 1 cup cranberries
- 1 cucumber
- 1 handful spinach
- 1 apple
- 1 cup pineapple

DIRECTIONS

1. **In a blender place all ingredients and blend until smooth**
2. **Pour smoothie in a glass and serve**

CITRUS FLUSH

Serves: *1*

Prep Time: *5* Minutes

Cook Time: *5* Minutes

Total Time: *10* Minutes

INGREDIENTS

- 1 orange
- 1 squeeze of lime
- 1 bunch of cilantro
- ¼ cup pineapple
- 1 stalk asparagus

DIRECTIONS

1. In a blender place all ingredients and blend until smooth
2. Pour smoothie in a glass and serve

NO MILK SHAKE

Serves: 1
Prep Time: 5 Minutes
Cook Time: 5 Minutes
Total Time: 10 Minutes

INGREDIENTS

- ½ cup pasteurized liquid egg product
- ¼ cup non-dairy whipped topping
- almond extract
- ½ cup berries
- vanilla extract

DIRECTIONS

1. In a blender place all ingredients and blend until smooth
2. Pour smoothie in a glass and serve

CHERRY SHAKE

Serves: **1**
Prep Time: **5** Minutes
Cook Time: **5** Minutes
Total Time: **10** Minutes

INGREDIENTS

- 1 cup tart cherries
- ½ avocado
- 1 tablespoon cacao powder
- stevia
- 2 tablespoons chia seeds
- ¼ tsp vanilla extract
- 100 ml almond milk

DIRECTIONS

1. In a blender place all ingredients and blend until smooth
2. Pour smoothie in a glass and serve

GOJI SMOOTHIE

Serves: *1*

Prep Time: *5* Minutes

Cook Time: *5* Minutes

Total Time: *10* Minutes

INGREDIENTS

- Zest of 1 orange
- 1 orange
- 1 banana
- ½ cup goji berries
- 1 tablespoon hemp seeds
- 1 tablespoon chia seeds
- ice cubes

DIRECTIONS

1. In a blender place all ingredients and blend until smooth
2. Pour smoothie in a glass and serve

ACAI SMOOTHIE

Serves: *1*
Prep Time: *5* Minutes
Cook Time: *5* Minutes
Total Time: *10* Minutes

INGREDIENTS

- 1 pack Acai puree
- 1 avocado
- 1 cup spinach
- 1 tablespoon chia seeds
- 1 tablespoon hemp hearts
- 1 pinch of stevia

DIRECTIONS

1. In a blender place all ingredients and blend until smooth
2. Pour smoothie in a glass and serve

MATCHA TEA SMOOTHIE

Serves: *1*

Prep Time: *5* Minutes

Cook Time: *5* Minutes

Total Time: *10* Minutes

INGREDIENTS

- 2 tsp Matcha
- ¼ cup spinach
- ½ avocado
- ½ banana
- ½ cup coconut water
- ½ cup orange juice

DIRECTIONS

1. In a blender place all ingredients and blend until smooth
2. Pour smoothie in a glass and serve

PUMPKIN PIE SMOOTHIE

Serves: *1*

Prep Time: *5* Minutes

Cook Time: *5* Minutes

Total Time: *10* Minutes

INGREDIENTS

- ½ cup pumpkin
- 1 cup unsweetened coconut milk
- ½ cup plain yogurt
- 1 tablespoon peanut butter
- ½ tsp pumpkin pie spice

DIRECTIONS

1. In a blender place all ingredients and blend until smooth
2. Pour smoothie in a glass and serve

ALMOND SMOOTHIE

Serves: **1**
Prep Time: **5** Minutes
Cook Time: **5** Minutes
Total Time: **10** Minutes

INGREDIENTS

- 1 cup sweet cherries
- 1 cup unsweetened almond milk
- 1 tablespoon butter
- 1tablespoon oats

DIRECTIONS

1. In a blender place all ingredients and blend until smooth
2. Pour smoothie in a glass and serve

DECAF VANILLA TEA LATTE

Serves: *1*

Prep Time: *5* Minutes

Cook Time: *0* Minutes

Total Time: *5* Minutes

INGREDIENTS

- ¼ Tsp coconut nectar
- Cinnamon

- 1 decaf vanilla tea bag
- ½ cup boiling water
- ½ cup coconut milk

DIRECTIONS

1. Steep tea in boiling water for 5 minutes.
2. Heat up the coconut milk in the microwave for 45 seconds.
3. Froth the coconut milk, then add to the steeped tea.
4. Add the coconut nectar and mix.
5. Top off with cinnamon.

GASTROPARESIS COOKBOOK

40+ Side Dishes, Salad and Pasta recipes designed for Gastroparesis

PASTA

LEMON PASTA

Serves: 2

Prep Time: *10* Minutes

Cook Time: *20* Minutes

Total Time: *30* Minutes

INGREDIENTS

- 2 handful of dry pasta
- 1 tablespoon cream cheese
- ¼ tsp salt
- 2 cups vegetable stock
- 1 lemon
- 1 handful basil

DIRECTIONS

1. In a saucepan add all the ingredients and cook over medium heat for 10-15 minutes
2. Stir frequently and add lemon slices and basil
3. Remove and serve

CHICKEN NOODLE SOUP

Serves: **4**

Prep Time: **10** Minutes

Cook Time: **40** Minutes

Total Time: **50** Minutes

INGREDIENTS

- 1 tsp olive oil
- 1 lb. chicken thighs
- 1 onion
- 2 ribs celery

- 2 carrots
- 2 cups chicken broths
- black pepper
- ¼ dried tarragon
- 3-quarts water
- 5-ounces noodles
- 1 tablespoon fresh parsley

DIRECTIONS

1. In a saucepan add one olive oil over medium heat
2. Add chicken and cook on low heat and remove it
3. Add onion, celery and cook for 5-10 minutes
4. Add carrots, chicken stock, chicken, tarragon and water
5. Reduce the heat and simmer for 40-45 minutes
6. Let it boil for 5-10 minutes and add noodles
7. Drain the noodles and serve with parsley

PASTA WITH NETTLE PESTO

Serves: *3*
Prep Time: *10* Minutes
Cook Time: *20* Minutes
Total Time: *30* Minutes

INGREDIENTS

- **1 cup nettle leaves**
- **½ cup parmesan cheese**
- **½ cup olive oil**
- **10 oz. pasta**
- **3 garlic cloves**
- **½ cup walnuts**

DIRECTIONS

1. In a food processor add garlic, walnuts, and leaves
2. Blend until smooth and olive oil and stir in parmesan cheese
3. Cook pasta and drain it
4. Sit in nettle pesto
5. Transfer onto serving plates and garnish with salt

CHICKEN PASTA

Serves: *4*

Prep Time: *10* Minutes

Cook Time: *30* Minutes

Total Time: *40* Minutes

INGREDIENTS

- 2 cups butternut squash
- 1 tablespoon olive oil
- 2 pieces of bacon
- 2 chicken breasts
- ¼ coconut cream
- 1 tablespoon apple cider vinegar

- 1 tablespoon coconut oil
- 1 tsp salt
- 1 tsp garlic powder
- 1 zucchini

DIRECTIONS

1. Spiralize the zucchini into noodles and cook in olive oil
2. In a blender add coconut cream, coconut oil, squash, vinegar, salt, garlic powder and blend until smooth
3. Pour the mixture over the noodles and toss to coat
4. Serve when ready

PASTA WITH BEEF

Serves: **4**

Prep Time: **10** Minutes

Cook Time: **2h 50** Minutes

Total Time: **3h** Minutes

INGREDIENTS

- 1-pound lean beef
- ¼ cup onion
- 3 cloves garlic
- 2 cans tomatoes
- 1 6-ounces can tomato paste
- 2 anchovy fillets
- 1 tsp oregano
- ½ tsp red pepper

- 6-ounces penne pasta
- 1/3 cup olives
- ½ cup parsley

DIRECTIONS

1. In a skillet add onion, garlic, and beef and cook on medium heat
2. In a slow cooker combine the beef mixture with anchovies, oregano, tomato paste, and red pepper
3. Cook for 5-6 hours
4. When ready, stir olives and parsley in the cooker
5. When ready remove and serve with parsley

SATAY NOODLES

Serves: *3*

Prep Time: *10* Minutes

Cook Time: *20* Minutes

Total Time: *30* Minutes

INGREDIENTS

- **2 courgettes spiralized**
- **¼ butternut squash**
- **Satay**
- **2 tablespoons coconut oil**
- **150g peanut butter**
- **1 can coconut milk**
- **1 tsp fish sauce**
- **1 onion**
- **1 chilli**

DIRECTIONS

1. Cut chicken into bite-size cubes and mix with chili, coconut oil, soy sauce, garlic and marinade
2. In a pan heat coconut oil and add chili and onion
3. Add chicken and cook until brown
4. Add peanut butter, fish sauce, and coconut milk and stir on low heat
5. Add noodles and cook until ready
6. Remove and serve with coriander

ZITI WITH MEAT SAUCE

Serves: 2

Prep Time: **10** Minutes

Cook Time: **50** Minutes

Total Time: **60** Minutes

INGREDIENTS

- **1-pound lean beef**
- **1 tablespoon fresh basil**
- **1 tsp onion powder**
- **1 tsp garlic powder**
- **1 cup mozzarella cheese**
- **1 cup carrot**
- **2 cans tomato soup**
- **2 cups water**
- **6-ounces ziti pasta**
- **½ cup Parmesan cheese**

DIRECTIONS

1. Cook beef with carrot over medium heat in a Dutch oven
2. Stir water, ziti, basil, tomato soup, garlic, and onion powder over in the oven
3. Let it boil and cook for 25-30 minutes until tender
4. Stir in mozzarella and sprinkle Parmesan cheese

NOODLE SOUP

Serves: **1**

Prep Time: **10** Minutes

Cook Time: **20** Minutes

Total Time: **30** Minutes

INGREDIENTS

- 2 cups water
- ¼ tsp ginger
- 1 cup bok choy
- 1 red pepper
- 1 tsp soy sauce
- 1 clove garlic
- ½ tsp spice powder
- 1 ounce somen noodles
- 1 cup cooked chicken
- 1 cup chicken broth
- 2 onions

DIRECTIONS

1. In a saucepan mix all the ingredients and bring to boil
2. Stir the mixture for 5-10 minutes after boiling
3. Remove from heat and let it cook
4. Serve hot

SALAD

MORNING SALAD

Serves: **2**

Prep Time: **5** Minutes

Cook Time: **5** Minutes

Total Time: **10** Minutes

INGREDIENTS

- **1 onion**
- **1 tsp cumin**
- **1 tablespoon olive oil**
- **1 avocado**
- **¼ lb. cooked lentils**
- **1 oz. walnuts**
- **Coriander**
- **¼ lb. feta cheese**
- **Salad dressing of choice**
- **8-10 baby carrots**

DIRECTIONS

1. In a bowl combine all ingredients together and mix well
2. Add dressing and serve

COLESLAW

Serves: 2
Prep Time: 5 Minutes
Cook Time: 5 Minutes
Total Time: 10 Minutes

INGREDIENTS

- 2 cabbage
- 2 carrot
- 1 apple
- 1 green onion
- ½ cup almonds
- ½ cup cranberries

DRESSING

- ½ cup Greek yogurt
- ¼ cup mayonnaise
- ¼ cup honey
- 1 tablespoon apple cider vinegar

DIRECTIONS

1. In a bowl combine all ingredients together and mix well

2. In another bowl prepare salad dressing
3. Combine salad with dressing and serve

ASIAN BROCCOLI SALAD

Serves: **6**

Prep Time: **5** Minutes

Cook Time: **5** Minutes

Total Time: **10** Minutes

INGREDIENTS

- 1 head broccoli
- 1 cup cooked edamame
- ¼ cup green onions
- ¼ cup peanuts
- 1 cup peanut sauce
- Sesame seeds

DIRECTIONS

1. In a bowl combine all ingredients together and mix well
2. In another bowl prepare salad dressing
3. Combine salad with dressing and serve

GRILLED EGGPLANT AND FETA SALAD

Serves: 2

Prep Time: 5 Minutes

Cook Time: 5 Minutes

Total Time: 10 Minutes

INGREDIENTS

- 2 Asian eggplants
- 1 tsp olive oil
- 1 cup tomatoes
- ¼ cup crumbled feta
- Salad dressing
- Seasoning

DIRECTIONS

1. In a bowl combine all ingredients together and mix well
2. In another bowl prepare salad dressing
3. Combine salad with dressing and serve

SHRIMP AND AVOCADO SALAD

Serves: **4**

Prep Time: **5** Minutes

Cook Time: **20** Minutes

Total Time: **25** Minutes

INGREDIENTS

- 1 cup shrimp
- 1 tablespoon chili oil
- ¼ tsp salt
- 1 avocado
- 1 grapefruit
- 1 cup rice
- ¼ cup balsamic reduction

DIRECTIONS

1. In a bowl combine all ingredients together and mix well
2. In another bowl prepare salad dressing
3. Combine salad with dressing and serve

KALE SALAD WITH CITRUS-MAPLE VINAIGRETTE

Serves: **8**

Prep Time: **10** Minutes

Cook Time: **45** Minutes

Total Time: **55** Minutes

INGREDIENTS

- 1 squash
- 2 tablespoons olive oil
- Salt
- ¼ cup orange juice
- 1 tablespoon wine vinegar
- 1 tablespoon maple syrup
- Zest from 1 orange
- 2 bunches kale leaves
- ¼ cup pomegranate seeds
- ¼ cup berries

DIRECTIONS

1. In a bowl combine all ingredients together and mix well
2. In another bowl prepare salad dressing
3. Combine salad with dressing and serve

GRILLED CORN SALAD

Serves: 6
Prep Time: 10 Minutes
Cook Time: 50 Minutes
Total Time: 60 Minutes

INGREDIENTS

- 2 cobs corn
- ½ tsp salt
- ½ tsp pepper
- ½ tsp cilantro
- ½ cup avocado
- 1 tablespoon red onion

DIRECTIONS

1. In a bowl combine all ingredients together and mix well
2. In another bowl prepare salad dressing
3. Combine salad with dressing and serve

SIDE DISHES

AVOCADO TOAST

Serves: 2
Prep Time: **10** Minutes
Cook Time: **15** Minutes
Total Time: **25** Minutes

INGREDIENTS

- ¼ lb. peas
- 1 avocado
- Juice of ½ lemon
- 3 oz. feta cheese
- 1 tsp mint
- 2 eggs
- 1 tsp wine vinegar

DIRECTIONS

1. Place the peas in a pan with water and cook for 4-5 minutes
2. In a blender add cooked peas, avocado, lime juice and blend for 1 minute
3. Add feta cheese, mint and blend for another 2-3 minutes
4. When ready spread on 2-3 bread slices and serve with poached eggs

VEGGIE BURGERS

Serves: **4**
Prep Time: **5** Minutes
Cook Time: **15** Minutes

Total Time: **20** Minutes

INGREDIENTS

- 1 lb. beef
- 1 carrot
- 1 zucchini
- 3 cloves garlic
- ¼ cup parsley
- 1 tablespoon parmesan
- 1 tablespoon coconut oil

DIRECTIONS

1. Grate zucchini and carrots in a bowl
2. In a pan melt coconut oil, add garlic, carrots, parsley, zucchini, pepper, salt and sauté for 2-3 minutes
3. Combine vegetables with beef, parmesan, mix and form patties
4. Grill the patties for 3-4 minutes per side
5. When ready remove and serve

BROCCOLI SOUP

Serves: 2
Prep Time: 5 Minutes
Cook Time: 15 Minutes
Total Time: 20 Minutes

INGREDIENTS

- 1 tablespoon olive oil
- ½ onion
- 1 cup broccoli florets
- 1 cup cauliflower
- 1 cup bone broth
- ¼ cup coconut milk
- 1 tsp salt

DIRECTIONS

1. Heat a pot over low heat, add garlic, broccoli, cauliflower, bone broth, coconut milk and cook on low heat until tender
2. In a blender transfer cooked vegetables and blend until smooth
3. When ready serve with chives on top

CRISPY DRUMSTICKS

Serves: 1
Prep Time: 5 Minutes
Cook Time: 5 Minutes
Total Time: 10 Minutes

INGREDIENTS

- 8 chicken drumsticks
- 1 tablespoon olive oil
- 1 tsp salt
- 1 tsp garlic
- 1 onion
- 1lb. figs
- 1 tablespoon chives

DIRECTIONS

1. Place drumsticks in a baking dish and drizzle olive oil, garlic powder, salt and bake for 90 minutes at 350 F
2. In the last 15-20 minutes, add onion, olive oil to a saucepan and cook until tender
3. Add balsamic vinegar, figs, salt, and chopped chives
4. When the drumsticks are done, remove and spoon the of the fig sauce over the drumsticks

BROILED SALMON

Serves: **4**

Prep Time: **5** Minutes

Cook Time: **15** Minutes

Total Time: **20** Minutes

INGREDIENTS

- **4 salmon fillets**

- 2 tablespoons olive oil
- 1 tsp salt

DIRECTIONS

1. Pat dry salmon fillets and sprinkle with salt and olive oil
2. Place in oven on the top rack and broil for 12-15 minutes
3. When done, add sliced lemon and serve

ROASTED ASPARAGUS

Serves: *4*

Prep Time: *5* Minutes

Cook Time: *10* Minutes

Total Time: *15* Minutes

INGREDIENTS

- 1 lb. asparagus
- 1 tablespoon olive oil
- 2 garlic cloves

- 2 tablespoons parmesan
- Juice of 1 lemon

DIRECTIONS

1. On a baking sheet arrange the asparagus and toss in the olive oil
2. Sprinkle with salt and pepper
3. Roast for 10-12 minutes or until tender
4. Toss in garlic, parmesan and lemon juice
5. When ready remove and serve

POTATO & CAULIFLOWER MASH

Serves: 2
Prep Time: 5   Minutes
Cook Time: 15   Minutes
Total Time: 20   Minutes

INGREDIENTS

- 1 lb. sweet potatoes
- 1 lb. cauliflower florets
- 2 tablespoons milk
- ¼ cup Greek Yogurt

- ¼ tsp garlic powder
- Salt

DIRECTIONS

1. Cut sweet potato into 1-inch cubes
2. In a pot steam sweet potato, add cauliflower, water, and steam for 12-15 minutes
3. In a bowl mass the potato, cauliflower and mix with milk
4. Stir in Greek yogurt, pepper, and garlic powder
5. When ready garnish with parsley

ROASTED BEETS

Serves: 6
Prep Time: 15 Minutes
Cook Time: 45 Minutes
Total Time: 60 Minutes

INGREDIENTS

- 4 beets
- 1 tsp salt
- 1 tablespoon olive oil
- 1 tablespoon maple syrup

DIRECTIONS

1. Cut the beets in 1-inch cubes
2. Place the beets on a baking sheet and toss with salt and olive oil
3. Roast for 30-40 minutes at 375 F
4. In a pan add maple syrup, vinegar and cook until liquid is evaporated
5. Toss the glaze with the roasted beets and serve

BAKED ZUCCHINI FRIES

Serves: **6-8**

Prep Time: **5** Minutes

Cook Time: **25** Minutes

Total Time: **30** Minutes

INGREDIENTS

- 2 zucchinis
- ¼ cup flour
- ¼ tsp salt
- ½ tsp garlic powder

- ½ cup milk
- 1 cup breadcrumbs

DIRECTIONS

1. Grease a rack and place it on a baking tray
2. Combine milk, spices, flour, and breadcrumbs
3. Dip each zucchini stick in flour mixture and place on the rack
4. Bake for 18-20 minutes
5. When ready remove and serve

CAULIFLOWER FRIED RICE

Serves: 2
Prep Time: 5 Minutes
Cook Time: 15 Minutes
Total Time: 20 Minutes

INGREDIENTS

- 1 cauliflower
- 1 tablespoon sesame oil
- 1 carrot
- 1 garlic clove

- 1 cup edamame
- 2 eggs
- 2 tablespoons soy sauce
- 4 green onions

DIRECTIONS

1. Shred cauliflower using a grater and blend until smooth
2. In a skillet heat sesame oil, add garlic, carrots and fry for 5-6 minutes
3. Add edamame, cauliflower and cook until soft
4. Add the eggs and stir in the soy sauce and green onions
5. When ready remove from heat and serve

TABBOULEH

Serves: 2
Prep Time: 5 Minutes
Cook Time: 15 Minutes
Total Time: 20 Minutes

INGREDIENTS

- 1 cup bulghur
- 1 cup boiling water
- ¼ cup olive oil
- 1 tsp salt
- 1 tsp pepper
- 1 cup cherry tomatoes

- 1 cup cucumber
- 1 cup green onions
- 1 cup mint leaves
- 1 cup parsley

DIRECTIONS

1. In a bowl add bulghur, boiling water, lemon juice, pepper, olive oil, salt, cover and set aside for one hour
2. Add remaining ingredients and stir to combine
3. Add seasoning and mix well
4. When ready serve and refrigerate

RED POTATOES & LEEKS

Serves: 2

Prep Time: 5 Minutes

Cook Time: 15 Minutes

Total Time: 20 Minutes

INGREDIENTS

- 1 lb. red potatoes
- 1 tablespoon olive oil
- 2 leeks
- ½ cup soy milk
- Salt

DIRECTIONS

1. In a saucepan bring water to a boil, add red potatoes and simmer for 12-15 minutes
2. In a skillet add leeks, sauté until soft and set aside
3. In a bowl combine soymilk with potatoes and using a potato masher, mash potatoes
4. Fold in leeks, season and serve

ROASTED CARROTS

Serves: 6
Prep Time: 5 Minutes
Cook Time: 25 Minutes
Total Time: 30 Minutes

INGREDIENTS

- 2 lbs. carrots
- 2 tablespoons olive oil
- 1 tablespoon maple syrup
- 1 tablespoon honey
- 1 tsp coriander
- 1 tsp salt
- ½ tsp black pepper
- 1 tablespoon sesame seeds

- 1 tablespoon thyme leaves
- 1 tablespoon chives

DIRECTIONS

1. In a pan add carrots, maple syrup, honey, and drizzle olive oil
2. Sprinkle coriander, salt and toss to coat
3. Roast carrots for 20-25 minutes
4. When ready remove, sprinkle sesame seeds over carrots and serve

OAT PORRIDGE

Serves: 1
Prep Time: 5 Minutes
Cook Time: 15 Minutes
Total Time: 20 Minutes

INGREDIENTS

- 1 oz. oats
- 200 ml coconut milk
- 2 tsp sunflower seeds
- 1 tsp vanilla sugar

DIRECTIONS

1. In a saucepan add oats, water and bring to a boil
2. Reduce heat and simmer for 5-10 minutes
3. In a pan add sunflower seeds and roast for 4-5 minutes

4. Stir in oats mixture roasted sunflower seeds, milk, sugar and mix well
5. Top with fruits and serve

GUACAMOLE WITH PISTACHIOS

Serves: 2
Prep Time: 5 Minutes
Cook Time: 10 Minutes
Total Time: 15 Minutes

INGREDIENTS

- 2 avocados
- 1 tablespoon lime juice
- 1 tablespoon minced red onion
- 1 tablespoon cilantro
- 1 garlic clover
- 1 jalapeno Chile
- ¼ cup pistachios

DIRECTIONS

1. Slice avocados lengthwise
2. Mash with onion, lime juice, garlic, cilantro, and jalapenos

3. Mix it with guacamole and mustachios
4. Sprinkle with salt, seasoning and mix well
5. Serve with tortilla chips

BAKED GREEN BEAN FRIES

Serves: **4**

Prep Time: **5** Minutes

Cook Time: **15** Minutes

Total Time: **20** Minutes

INGREDIENTS

- 1 lb. green beans
- 2 eggs
- 1 cup breadcrumbs
- 1 tsp garlic powder
- ½ tsp paprika
- Sriracha sauce

DIRECTIONS

1. In a bowl add garlic, paprika, panko and set aside
2. In another bowl add eggs and whisk well
3. Add green beans in the egg mixture and fold in panko mixture

4. Bake for 12-15 minutes at 440 F or until crispy
5. When ready, serve with sriracha sauce

COCONUT PINEAPPLE CASHEW RICE

Serves: **4**

Prep Time: **5** Minutes

Cook Time: **25** Minutes

Total Time: **30** Minutes

INGREDIENTS

- 1 cup cooked rice
- 1 can pineapple juice
- 1 can unsweetened coconut milk
- 2 tablespoons coconut flakes
- 1 tablespoon red curry paste
- 1 tsp garlic powder
- ¼ tsp onion powder
- ¼ tsp salt

DIRECTIONS

1. Drain a can of crushed pineapple, add coconut milk, water and pour into a saucepan

2. Bring to a simmer stir in remaining ingredients
3. Simmer for 18-20 minutes
4. When ready remove and serve

GRILLED CORN

Serves: 2
Prep Time: 5 Minutes
Cook Time: 15 Minutes
Total Time: 20 Minutes

INGREDIENTS

- 2 ears corn
- ¼ cup mayonnaise
- 1 cup sour cream
- ½ cup cilantro
- 1 cup parmesan
- 1 lime

DIRECTIONS

1. Grill the corn for 4-5 minutes per side
2. In a bowl combine sour cream, cilantro and mayonnaise

3. When ready remove from corn the grill and slather with the mayonnaise mixture
4. Serve with lime juice and parmesan

VEGETABLE KABOBS

Serves: **4**
Prep Time: **5** Minutes
Cook Time: **15** Minutes
Total Time: **20** Minutes

INGREDIENTS

- 2 cups cremini mushrooms
- 1 cup cherry tomatoes
- 1 red bell pepper
- 1 green bell pepper
- 1 red onion
- 1 zucchini
- 1 yellow zucchini

MARINADE

- ½ cup olive oil
- 2 cloves garlic
- Juice of 1 lemon

- ¼ tsp oregano

DIRECTIONS

1. In a bowl whisk together lemon juice, oregano, basil, olive oil, garlic, salt and pepper
2. Thread tomatoes, mushrooms, bell peppers, onion, and zucchini onto skewers
3. Brush with olive oil mixture and roast for 12-15 minutes or until tender
4. When ready remove and serve

SQUASH FRIES

Serves: 3
Prep Time: 5 Minutes
Cook Time: 15 Minutes
Total Time: 20 Minutes

INGREDIENTS

- 1 butternut squash
- 1 tsp olive oil
- 1 tsp salt

DIRECTIONS

1. **Cut squash in thin slices**
2. **Place squash in a bowl and coat with olive oil**
3. **Sprinkle with salt and lay fries on baking sheets**
4. **Broil in the oven until crispy, when ready remove and serve**

ROASTED CAULIFLOWER

Serves: **4**

Prep Time: **5** Minutes

Cook Time: **25** Minutes

Total Time: **30** Minutes

INGREDIENTS

- 20 oz. cauliflower florets
- ½ cup coconut oil
- 2 cloves garlic
- Salt
- ¼ cup grated parmesan
- 1 tablespoon parsley leaves

DIRECTIONS

1. Place cauliflowers onto a baking sheet
2. Add garlic, coconut oil, salt, pepper and toss well
3. Bake for 20-25 minutes at 425 F
4. When ready remove and serve

BANANA SNAPS

Serves: **8**

Prep Time: **10** Minutes

Cook Time: **50** Minutes

Total Time: **60** Minutes

INGREDIENTS

- 1 cup pecan meal
- 3 cups almond flour
- ½ tsp salt
- ½ tsp baking soda
- 1 tsp cinnamon
- ½ cup ripe banana
- ¼ cup butter
- ¼ cup honey
- 1 egg
- 1 tsp vanilla extract
-

DIRECTIONS

1. In a bowl combine dry ingredients with wet ingredients, mix until fully incorporated
2. Place in the freezer for 20-30 minutes

3. Roll dough into balls and place on a cookie sheet
4. Bake for 22-25 minutes at 325 F
5. When ready remove and serve

GINGER SOUP

Serves: **4**

Prep Time: **5** Minutes

Cook Time: **20** Minutes

Total Time: **25** Minutes

INGREDIENTS

- 4 cups water
- 1 sheet nori
- 1 tsp grated ginger
- 4 tablespoons miso paste
- ½ cup green onion
- 2 baby bok choy
- 1 cup shiitake mushrooms
- ½ cup tofu
- Salt

DIRECTIONS

1. Bring water to a simmer
2. Add in nori and simmer for another 4-5 minutes
3. In another bowl add ½ cup water, miso paste and stir until miso dissolves completely

4. Add ginger, onion, bok choy, tofu, mushrooms, and simmer for 10-12 minutes
5. Remove pot from heat and stir in miso mixture
6. Stir well and taste
7. When ready pour into bowls and serve

ASIAN GREEN BEANS

Serves: 2
Prep Time: 5 Minutes
Cook Time: 15 Minutes
Total Time: 20 Minutes

INGREDIENTS

- 1 tablespoon sesame oil
- ½ tsp red pepper flakes
- 2 cloves garlic
- 1-inch piece ginger
- 8 oz. green beans
- 1 tablespoon coconut aminos
- 1 tablespoon wine vinegar
- 1 tsp honey

DIRECTIONS

1. In a wok add sesame oil, red pepper flakes, garlic, ginger and stir well
2. Add green beans, garlic, ginger and fry until tender
3. Pour in the wine vinegar, honey, coconut aminos and stir to combine

4. Simmer for 5-10 minutes or until tender
5. When ready remove from heat and serve

ZUCCHINI WITH BALSAMIC REDUCTION

Serves: **4**

Prep Time: **5** Minutes

Cook Time: **35** Minutes

Total Time: **40** Minutes

INGREDIENTS

- 2 tablespoons olive oil
- 2 zucchinis
- Salt
- Pepper
- ½ tsp paprika
- Sesame seeds
- Dried mint

BALSAMIC GLAZE

- 1 cup balsamic vinegar
- 1 tablespoon brown sugar

DIRECTIONS

1. In a saucepan, heat balsamic vinegar and sugar, bring to a boil and simmer for 18-20 minutes, when ready, remove from heat
2. In a skillet heat olive oil, add zucchini, salt, paprika, pepper and sauté for 5-10 minutes
3. When ready, transfer to a place, drizzle balsamic glaze and serve with sesame seeds on top

GASTROPARESIS COOKBOOK

40+ Smoothies, Dessert and Breakfast recipes designed for Gastroparesis

BREAKFAST

CHIA SEEDS WITH MAPLE SYRUP

Serves: **1**

Prep Time: **10** Minutes

Cook Time: **8** Hours

Total Time: **8** Hours

INGREDIENTS

- 2 tablespoons chia seeds
- 1 tablespoon oats
- 250 ml almond milk
- 2 pecan nuts
- 1 tsp maple syrup
- 2 oz. raspberries

DIRECTIONS

1. In a bowl combine all ingredients together
2. Leave in the fridge overnight
3. Serve in the morning

COURGETTE SHAKSHUKA

Serves: 2
Prep Time: 5 Minutes
Cook Time: 10 Minutes
Total Time: 15 Minutes

INGREDIENTS

- 2 big Courgettes
- 2 tablespoons olive oil
- 2 tablespoons sunflower seeds
- 2 cloves garlic
- 12 cherry tomatoes
- Juice from ¼ lemon
- 4 eggs

DIRECTIONS

1. Cut each courgette and spiralize them
2. Place the spiraled courgettes in a pan and cook on low heat for 5-10 minutes
3. Add the eggs on top, cover with a lid and cook for 4-5 minutes
4. When ready sprinkle with parsley, seasoning and serve

MORNING SALAD

Serves: 2

Prep Time: 5 Minutes

Cook Time: 5 Minutes

Total Time: 10 Minutes

INGREDIENTS

- 1 onion
- 1 tsp cumin
- 1 tablespoon olive oil
- 1 avocado
- ¼ lb. cooked lentils
- 1 oz. walnuts
- Coriander
- ¼ lb. feta cheese
- Salad dressing of choice
- 8-10 baby carrots

DIRECTIONS

1. In a bowl combine all ingredients together and mix well
2. Add dressing and serve

AVOCADO TOAST

Serves: 2

Prep Time: 10 Minutes

Cook Time: 15 Minutes

Total Time: 25 Minutes

INGREDIENTS

- ¼ lb. peas
- 1 avocado
- Juice of ½ lemon
- 3 oz. feta cheese
- 1 tsp mint
- 2 eggs
- 1 tsp wine vinegar

DIRECTIONS

1. In a blender add cooked peas, avocado, lime juice and blend for 1 minute
2. Add feta cheese, mint and blend for another 2-3 minutes
3. When ready spread on 2-3 bread slices and serve with poached eggs

GLUTEN-FREE BREAD

Serves: **8**

Prep Time: **10** Minutes

Cook Time: **3** Hours

Total Time: **3** Hours and 10 Minutes

INGREDIENTS

- ¼ lb. rice flour
- ¼ lb. buckwheat flour
- ¼ lb. gluten-free almond flour
- 1 tsp salt
- 2 oz. sunflower seeds
- 2 oz. pumpkin seeds
- 1 oz. sesame seeds
- 400 ml water

DIRECTIONS

1. In a bowl combine all ingredients together
2. Mix well using a wooden spoon and cover for 1-2 hours
3. Transfer the mixture to the loaf tin

4. Place the bread in the oven and cook at 400 F for 25-30 minutes
5. When ready remove and serve

SAGE PATE

Serves: 2

Prep Time: 5 Minutes

Cook Time: 5 Minutes

Total Time: 10 Minutes

INGREDIENTS

- 100 g tomato
- 100 g walnuts
- 1 tablespoon sage leaves
- salt

DIRECTIONS

1. Place all ingredients in a blender and blend until smooth
2. Season pate with salt and pepper
3. Spread the pate on toast and serve

BANANA MUFFINS

Serves: *12*
Prep Time: *10* Minutes
Cook Time: *30* Minutes
Total Time: *40* Minutes

INGREDIENTS

- 1 cup almond flour
- 1 cup pecan pieces
- 1 tsp cinnamon
- ¼ tsp nutmeg
- ¼ tsp baking powder
- ½ tsp salt
- 2 bananas
- 1 tablespoon honey
- 2 eggs

DIRECTIONS

1. Preheat the oven to 400 F
2. In a food processor add pecan pieces, cinnamon, almond flour, nutmeg, baking powder, salt and process for 45-60 seconds

3. Mush bananas, add honey, eggs and mix well
4. Add the flour mixture to the egg mixture and mix well
5. Scoop the batter into 12 muffin cups
6. Bake for 22-25 minutes or until ready

KEDGEREE WITH TURMERIC

Serves: 2

Prep Time: 10 Minutes

Cook Time: 30 Minutes

Total Time: 40 Minutes

INGREDIENTS

- 2 tablespoons olive oil
- ¼ tsp turmeric
- Grated ginger
- 1/3 lb. basmati rice
- 4 eggs
- ½ lb. haddock
- salt
- coriander leaves

DIRECTIONS

1. In a pan add ginger, turmeric, rice and water
2. Bring to a boil and simmer for 15-20 minutes or until the rice is ready, cover with a lid
3. Add haddock and cook for another 5-6 minutes
4. Boil eggs for 5-10 minutes scatter coriander over the kedgeree and serve

SUNFLOWER SEED PATE

Serves: 2

Prep Time: 5 Minutes

Cook Time: 10 Minutes

Total Time: 15 Minutes

INGREDIENTS

- 2 red peppers
- 3 oz. sunflower seeds
- Pinch of paprika
- Salt
- Juice ½ lemon
- 1 tsp rosemary

DIRECTIONS

1. Place the peppers on a baking tray and roast for 30 minutes at 375 F
2. Place the sunflower seeds on another baking tray and bake for 5-6 minutes
3. Place the peppers, paprika, lemon juice, sunflower seeds and rosemary in a blender and blend until smooth
4. Spread pate on toast and serve

WHITEBAIT FRITTERS

Serves: **6**

Prep Time: **10** Minutes

Cook Time: **15** Minutes

Total Time: **25** Minutes

INGREDIENTS

- 2/3 lb. whitebait
- 2 eggs
- 1 clove garlic
- herbs (onions, mint, basil, etc)
- 1 tablespoon olive oil

DIRECTIONS

1. In a bowl combine all ingredients together
2. In a skillet heat olive oil and our batter
3. Fry for 2-3 minutes per side or until golden brown
4. When ready remove and serve

DESSERTS

PEARS POACHED WITH LEMON

Serves: 6
Prep Time: 5 Minutes
Cook Time: 30 Minutes
Total Time: 35 Minutes

INGREDIENTS

- 1 oz. hibiscus flowers
- Zest of one lemon
- ¼ lb. sugar
- 6 pears
- 1 L water

DIRECTIONS

1. Place the hibiscus flowers in a saucepan with lemon zest, sugar, water and bring to a boil
2. Simmer on low heat for 12-15 minutes until sugar is fully dissolved
3. Pour the liquid in a de7ep saucepan and dip the pears into the liquid, simmer for 10-15 minutes
4. When the pears are cooked remove them to a serving dish
5. The rest of the liquid bring to a boil until the liquid is mostly evaporated
6. Pour remaining liquid over pears and serve

BUTTER COOKIES

Serves: **12**

Prep Time: **5** Minutes

Cook Time: **15** Minutes

Total Time: **20** Minutes

INGREDIENTS

- 2 cups almond flour
- ¼ tsp salt
- ¼ tsp baking soda
- ¼ tsp butter
- 4 tablespoons honey
- 2 tsp vanilla extract

DIRECTIONS

1. Preheat the oven to 325 F
2. In a bowl combine dry ingredients with wet ingredients and mix until fully incorporated
3. Set aside for 50-60 minutes
4. Roll into small balls and press them on a cookie sheet
5. Bake for 10-12 minutes or until golden brown
6. When ready, remove and serve

FROZEN STRAWBERRY CAKE

Serves: 6
Prep Time: 5 Minutes
Cook Time: 5 Minutes

Total Time: *10* Minutes

INGREDIENTS

- 1 lb. sunflower seeds
- 12 medjool dates
- 1 tablespoon coconut oil
- 1 lb. strawberries
- Juice of ¼ lemon
- 1 lb. Greek yogurt

DIRECTIONS

1. Preheat the oven to 350 F
2. Place the sunflower seeds on a baking sheet and bake for 5-6 minutes
3. Place baked sunflower seeds in a blender and blend until smooth
4. Add coconut oil, dates, strawberries, lime juice, Greek yogurt and blend until
5. Pour mixture in the cake tin and place in the freezer for 2-3 hours
6. When ready remove, decorate and serve

MANGO AND LIME SORBET

Serves: 2
Prep Time: 5 Minutes
Cook Time: 5 Minutes
Total Time: 10 Minutes

INGREDIENTS

- 1 lb. mango
- 1 lime
- ¼ lb. coconut water
- 200 g berries
- ¼ lb. coconut shavings

DIRECTIONS

1. In a blender add mango, lime juice, zest, coconut water, and blend until smooth
2. When ready add berries, coconut shavings and serve

HONEY BAKED PLUMBS

Serves: *4*
Prep Time: *5* Minutes
Cook Time: *20* Minutes
Total Time: *25* Minutes

INGREDIENTS

- 4 red plumbs
- 2 tablespoons runny honey
- 1 tablespoon pistachio nuts
- 1 lb. labneh
- ½ lb. Greek yogurt
- Pinch of saffron
- 3 cardamom pods

DIRECTIONS

1. Preheat the oven to 350 F
2. Place the plumbs on a baking tray, drizzle with honey and bake for 12-15 minutes or until ready
3. Mix saffron with water and set aside for a couple of minutes
4. Fold together the labneh, cardamom and saffron water
5. Divide the plumbs among serving bowls, top with saffron labneh and sprinkle with pistachio nuts

PUMPKIN CARAMEL CAKE

Serves: *8*

Prep Time: *10* Minutes

Cook Time: *45* Minutes

Total Time: *55* Minutes

INGREDIENTS

- ¼ cup honey
- 1 cup pumpkin puree

- 2 sticks butter
- 4 eggs
- 1 cup almond flour
- ¼ tsp salt
- 1 tablespoon cinnamon
- ¼ tsp ginger
- ½ tsp nutmeg
- 1 tsp baking soda

DIRECTIONS

1. In a bowl mix all ingredients until fully incorporated
2. Pour into a greased cake pan
3. Bake at 375 F for 40-45 minutes
4. When ready, remove pour caramel sauce and serve

LIME YOGURT CAKE

Serves: **6**

Prep Time: **10** Minutes

Cook Time: **50** Minutes

Total Time: **60** Minutes

INGREDIENTS

- ¼ lb. butter
- ¼ lb. sugar
- 1 egg
- 2 oz. buckwheat flour

- 2 oz. flour
- 1 tsp baking powder
- 2 oz. almonds
- 2 tablespoons Greek Yogurt
- ¼ lb. raspberries
- 2 oz. hazelnuts
- 2 tsp poppy seeds

DIRECTIONS

1. Preheat the oven to 375 F
2. In a cake tin line a baking paper
3. In a bowl combine butter, sugar, egg, flour, baking powder, almonds and mix well
4. Add Greek Yogurt, poppy seeds, raspberries and mix again
5. Spoon the mixture in the cake tin and bake for 50-60 minutes
6. When ready remove and serve

OAT PORRIDGE

Serves: *1*
Prep Time: *5* Minutes
Cook Time: *15* Minutes
Total Time: *20* Minutes

INGREDIENTS

- 1 oz. oats
- 200 ml coconut milk
- 2 tsp sunflower seeds
- 1 tsp vanilla sugar

DIRECTIONS

1. In a saucepan add oats, water and bring to a boil
2. Reduce heat and simmer for 5-10 minutes
3. In a pan add sunflower seeds and roast for 4-5 minutes
4. Stir in oats mixture roasted sunflower seeds, milk, sugar and mix well
5. Top with fruits and serve

ALMOND PANCAKES

Serves: 4

Prep Time: 5 Minutes

Cook Time: 15 Minutes

Total Time: 20 Minutes

INGREDIENTS

- 1 cup almond flour
- ¼ cup rice flour
- ¼ cup sugar
- ¼ tsp salt
- 1 tsp baking powder
- 2 eggs

- 1 cup almond milk
- 1 tsp lemon zest
- ¼ cup almonds

DIRECTIONS

1. In a bowl combine all ingredients together and whisk to combine
2. Spoon ¼ batter and cook for 2-3 minutes per side
3. When ready remove and serve

BANANA SNAPS

Serves: 8
Prep Time: 10 Minutes
Cook Time: 50 Minutes
Total Time: 60 Minutes

INGREDIENTS

- 1 cup pecan meal
- 3 cups almond flour
- ½ tsp salt
- ½ tsp baking soda
- 1 tsp cinnamon

- ½ cup ripe banana
- ¼ cup butter
- ¼ cup honey
- 1 egg
- 1 tsp vanilla extract

DIRECTIONS

1. In a bowl combine dry ingredients with wet ingredients, mix until fully incorporated
2. Place in the freezer for 20-30 minutes
3. Roll dough into balls and place on a cookie sheet
4. Bake for 22-25 minutes at 325 F
5. When ready remove and serve

SMOOTHIES

BANANA BREAKFAST SMOOTHIE

Serves: **1**

Prep Time: **5** Minutes

Cook Time: **5** Minutes

Total Time: **10** Minutes

INGREDIENTS

- ½ cup vanilla yogurt
- 2 tsp honey
- Pinch of cinnamon
- 1 banana
- 1 cup ice

DIRECTIONS

1. In a blender place all ingredients and blend until smooth
2. Pour the smoothie in a glass and serve

STRAWBERRY SUMMER SMOOTHIE

Serves: 1

Prep Time: 5 Minutes

Cook Time: 5 Minutes

Total Time: 10 Minutes

INGREDIENTS

- 1 banana
- 1 cup strawberries
- ¼ cup Greek yogurt
- 1 tsp honey
- 1 pinch cinnamon
- 1 cup ice

DIRECTIONS

1. In a blender place all ingredients and blend until smooth
2. Pour the smoothie in a glass and serve

RASPBERRY-ORANGE SMOOTHIE

Serves: *1*

Prep Time: *5* Minutes

Cook Time: *5* Minutes

Total Time: *10* Minutes

INGREDIENTS

- 1 cup orange juice
- 1 cup raspberries
- ¼ cup yogurt
- 1 cup ice

DIRECTIONS

1. In a blender place all ingredients and blend until smooth

2. Pour the smoothie in a glass and serve

PEACH & MANGO SMOOTHIE

Serves: *1*
Prep Time: *5* Minutes
Cook Time: *5* Minutes
Total Time: *10* Minutes

INGREDIENTS

- 1 cup peaches
- 1 cup mango
- 1 cup yogurt
- ¼ banana
- 1 cup ice

DIRECTIONS

1. **In a blender place all ingredients and blend until smooth**

2. Pour the smoothie in a glass and serve

CARROT MILKSHAKE

Serves: *1*
Prep Time: *5* Minutes
Cook Time: *5* Minutes
Total Time: *10* Minutes

INGREDIENTS

- 1 cup carrots
- 1 cup coconut milk
- 1 cup protein powder
- 1-inch turmeric
- 1-inch ginger
- ¼ tsp cinnamon

DIRECTIONS

1. In a blender place all ingredients and blend until smooth
2. Pour the smoothie in a glass and serve

CARROT SMOOTHIE

Serves: 1
Prep Time: 5 Minutes
Cook Time: 5 Minutes
Total Time: 10 Minutes

INGREDIENTS

- 1 cup carrots
- 1 cup apple juice
- 1 cup almonds
- 1 cup ice

DIRECTIONS

1. In a blender place all ingredients and blend until smooth
2. Pour the smoothie in a glass and serve

CUCUMBER SMOOTHIE

Serves: *1*

Prep Time: *5* Minutes

Cook Time: *5* Minutes

Total Time: *10* Minutes

INGREDIENTS

- 1 cucumber
- 1 lime
- ½ cup water
- 1 cup ice
- 1 tsp sugar
- 1 tsp honey

DIRECTIONS

1. In a blender place all ingredients and blend until smooth
2. Pour the smoothie in a glass and serve

KIWI DETOX SMOOTHIE

Serves: *1*

Prep Time: *5* Minutes

Cook Time: *5* Minutes

Total Time: *10* Minutes

INGREDIENTS

- 1 cup strawberries
- 1 cup mango
- 2 kiwis
- 1 tablespoon sugar
- 1 cup ice
- 1 cup coconut milk

DIRECTIONS

1. In a blender place all ingredients and blend until smooth
2. Pour the smoothie in a glass and serve

CHERRY SMOOTHIE

Serves: **1**

Prep Time: **5** Minutes

Cook Time: **5** Minutes

Total Time: **10** Minutes

INGREDIENTS

- 1 cup cherries
- 1 cup coconut milk
- 2 tablespoons sugar
- ¼ tsp vanilla extract
- 1 cup ice

DIRECTIONS

1. **In a blender place all ingredients and blend until smooth**
2. **Pour the smoothie in a glass and serve**

MOCHA FAUXCCHINO

Serves: **1**

Prep Time: **5** Minutes

Cook Time: **5** Minutes

Total Time: **10** Minutes

INGREDIENTS

- 2 cups coffee
- 2 cups coconut milk
- 1 cup ice cubes
- whipped cream for topping
- caramel sauce

DIRECTIONS

1. **In a blender place all ingredients and blend until smooth**
2. **Pour the smoothie in a glass and serve**

ALMOND SMOOTHIE

Serves: **1**

Prep Time: **5** Minutes

Cook Time: **5** Minutes

Total Time: **10** Minutes

INGREDIENTS

- ½ cup almonds
- 1 cup apricot nectar
- ¼ cup apricots
- ¼ cup Greek yogurt
- 1 tablespoon almond butter
- 1 cup ice

DIRECTIONS

1. In a blender place all ingredients and blend until smooth
2. Pour the smoothie in a glass and serve

GRAPE SMOOTHIE

Serves: 1

Prep Time: 5 Minutes

Cook Time: 5 Minutes

Total Time: 10 Minutes

INGREDIENTS

- 2 cups grapes
- 1 cup grape juice
- 1 cup ice
- 1 cup coconut water
- Coconut flakes

DIRECTIONS

1. **In a blender place all ingredients and blend until smooth**
2. **Pour the smoothie in a glass and serve**

PEAR SMOOTHIE

Serves: **1**

Prep Time: **5** Minutes

Cook Time: **5** Minutes

Total Time: **10** Minutes

INGREDIENTS

- ½ cup blueberries
- 1 pear
- 1 cup maple syrup
- 1 cup Greek yogurt
- 1 cup ice
- 1 tsp sugar

DIRECTIONS

1. **In a blender place all ingredients and blend until smooth**
2. **Pour the smoothie in a glass and serve**

GRAPEFRUIT SMOOTHIE

Serves: *1*

Prep Time: *5* Minutes

Cook Time: *5* Minutes

Total Time: *10* Minutes

INGREDIENTS

- 1 grapefruit
- 2 tablespoons brown sugar
- 1 cup ice
- 1 pinch cinnamon
- 1 lime slice
- Grate ginger

DIRECTIONS

1. In a blender place all ingredients and blend until smooth
2. Pour the smoothie in a glass and serve

PUMPKIN DETOX SMOOTHIE

Serves: **1**

Prep Time: **5** Minutes

Cook Time: **5** Minutes

Total Time: **10** Minutes

INGREDIENTS

- 1 banana
- 1 big handful of spinach
- ½ cup pumpkin puree
- 1 cup coconut milk
- 1 tablespoon flax seed
- 1 cup ice cubes
- 1 pinch of cinnamon

DIRECTIONS

1. In a blender place all ingredients and blend until smooth
2. Pour the smoothie in a glass and serve

POMEGRANATE SMOOTHIE

Serves: 1
Prep Time: 5 Minutes
Cook Time: 5 Minutes
Total Time: 10 Minutes

INGREDIENTS

- 1 cup cherries
- 1 cup pomegranate juice
- ¼ tablespoon honey
- ¼ tsp maple syrup
- 1 pinch cinnamon
- 1 cup ice
- ¼ cup coconut water

DIRECTIONS

1. In a blender place all ingredients and blend until smooth
2. Pour the smoothie in a glass and serve

WATERMELON SMOOTHIE

Serves: **1**

Prep Time: **5** Minutes

Cook Time: **5** Minutes

Total Time: **10** Minutes

INGREDIENTS

- 2 cups watermelon
- 1 cup lime juice
- ¼ brown sugar
- 1 cup water
- ¼ cup coconut water
- 1 cup ice

DIRECTIONS

1. In a blender place all ingredients and blend until smooth
2. Pour the smoothie in a glass and serve

CELERY SMOOTHIE

Serves: *1*

Prep Time: *5* Minutes

Cook Time: *5* Minutes

Total Time: *10* Minutes

INGREDIENTS

- 1 cup cherries
- 1 cup beets
- 1 cup coconut milk
- 1 banana
- ¼ tsp cinnamon

DIRECTIONS

1. **In a blender place all ingredients and blend until smooth**
2. **Pour the smoothie in a glass and serve**

GINGER SMOOTHIE

Serves: **1**

Prep Time: **5** Minutes

Cook Time: **5** Minutes

Total Time: **10** Minutes

INGREDIENTS

- 1 apple
- ½ inch ginger
- 1 lime
- ¼ cup honey
- 1 cup water
- 1 cup ice

DIRECTIONS

1. In a blender place all ingredients and blend until smooth
2. Pour the smoothie in a glass and serve

KIWI SMOOTHIE 2

Serves: *1*

Prep Time: *5* Minutes

Cook Time: *5* Minutes

Total Time: *10* Minutes

INGREDIENTS

- 1 cup almond milk
- 2 kiwi fruits
- 1 banana
- ¼ tsp ginger

DIRECTIONS

1. **In a blender place all ingredients and blend until smooth**
2. **Pour the smoothie in a glass and serve**

GASTROPARESIS COOKBOOK

40+ Soup, pizza and side dishes recipes designed for Gastroparesis diet

SOUP RECIPES

CABBAGE SOUP

Serves: **6**

Prep Time: **5** Minutes

Cook Time: **50** Minutes

Total Time: **55** Minutes

INGREDIENTS

- **2 tablespoons olive oil**
- **1 onion**
- **1 celery stick**
- **1 carrot**
- **3 oz. pancetta**
- **1 cabbage**
- **2 garlic cloves**
- **1 tsp paprika**
- **1tsp rosemary**
- **1 lb. tomatoes**
- **2 L chicken broth**
- **1 can chickpeas**

DIRECTIONS

1. In a pot heat oil and add carrot, celery, onion, salt and cook until vegetables are soft
2. Add the cabbage, garlic, paprika, rosemary and cook for another 8-10 minutes
3. Add tomatoes, stock, chickpeas and bring to a simmer and cook for 30 minutes
4. When ready serve with parmesan cheese

LENTIL SOUP

Serves: *4*

Prep Time: *5* Minutes

Cook Time: *25* Minutes

Total Time: *30* Minutes

INGREDIENTS

- 2 tsp cumin seeds
- 2 tablespoons olive oil
- 1 ½ lb. carrots
- ¼ lb. red lentils
- 1 L vegetable stock
- ¼ lb. milk

DIRECTIONS

1. In a saucepan fry, cumin seeds for 1-2 minutes
2. Add olive oil, carrots, vegetable stock, red lentils, stock, milk and bring to a boil
3. Simmer for 18-20 minutes
4. When ready blend the soup and pour in serving dishes
5. Sprinkle with spices and serve

PUMPKIN SOUP

Serves: **6**

Prep Time: **5** Minutes

Cook Time: **35** Minutes

Total Time: **40** Minutes

INGREDIENTS

- 2 tablespoons olive oil
- 2 onions
- 1 kg pumpkin
- 1 ½ lb. vegetable stock
- ¼ lb. double cream
- croutons

DIRECTIONS

1. In a saucepan cook onions for 5-6 minutes, add pumpkin, vegetable stock, salt and bring to a boil, simmer for 20-25 minutes
2. Add double cream and cook for another 8-10 minutes
3. When ready puree the soup and serve with croutons

MUSHROOM SOUP

Serves: **6**

Prep Time: **5** Minutes

Cook Time: **35** Minutes

Total Time: **40** Minutes

INGREDIENTS

- 1 tablespoon olive oil
- 1 onion
- 1 oz. mushrooms
- 2 tablespoons bouillon powder
- 1 lb. chestnut mushrooms
- 1 lb. potato
- 1 tsp thyme
- 2 carrots
- 1 tablespoon parsley
- 4 tablespoons Greek yogurt

DIRECTIONS

1. In a pan fry, onions until golden, add boiling water, mushrooms bouillon and continue to cook

2. Add the rest of the mushrooms, garlic, potatoes, carrots, thyme and continue to cook until vegetables are soft
3. Simmer for 20-25 minutes, stir in parsley and pepper
4. When ready remove from heat and serve with Greek Yogurt

LEEK SOUP

Serves: **4**

Prep Time: **5** Minutes

Cook Time: **25** Minutes

Total Time: **30** Minutes

INGREDIENTS

- 1 tablespoon oil
- 1 lb. leeks
- 1 lb. courgettes
- 2 tsp bouillon powder
- 1 lb. spinach
- ¼ lb. goat cheese
- 1 oz. basil

DIRECTIONS

1. In a pan, fry leeks until soft, add the courgettes, stock, bouillon powder, and cook for 12-15 minutes
2. Add spinach, goat's cheese, basil and cover the pan, cook for 8-10 minutes or until vegetables are soft
3. When ready remove from heat, add extra basil if necessary and serve

BUTTERNUT SQUASH SOUP

Serves: **6**

Prep Time: **10** Minutes

Cook Time: **40** Minutes

Total Time: **50** Minutes

INGREDIENTS

- 1 butternut squash
- 1 tablespoon olive oil
- 1 tablespoon butter
- 1 onion
- 1 garlic clove
- 2 lbs. low-sodium vegetable stock
- 2 tablespoons crème Fraiche

DIRECTIONS

1. Preheat oven to 375 F
2. Cut the butternut squash into cubes and toss with olive oil
3. Roast for 20-30 minutes or until golden brown
4. In a saucepan melt butter, add onions and garlic
5. Cook for 8-10 minutes or until onions are soft
6. Add vegetable stock and crème Fraiche to the butternut squash and mix well

7. Blend the mixture until smooth and pour to the pan
8. When ready, season to taste and serve with chili

OXTAIL SOUP

Serves: **6**

Prep Time: **10** Minutes

Cook Time: **4** Hours

Total Time: **4** Hours 10 Minutes

INGREDIENTS

- 3 lb. oxtail
- 2 bay leaves
- Parsley
- ¼ tsp black peppercorns
- ½ bottle red wine
- 3 tablespoons olive oil
- 2 carrots
- 2 celery sticks
- 2 garlic cloves
- 1 tablespoon plain flour
- 1 tablespoon ketchup
- A handful of thyme springs
- 2 L chicken stock

DIRECTIONS

1. Tie the bay leaves, thyme sprigs, parsley and put in the bowl with the peppercorns

2. Add wine, oxtail and cover overnight
3. Remove oxtail from marinade and transfer to a pan
4. Add carrots, celery, onion, garlic, flour, ketchup and cook until thickens
5. Pour over the marinade and simmer for a couple of minutes
6. Add stock and bring to a boil
7. When ready transfer to the oven at cook for 3-4 hours at 300 F or until the meat is tender
8. When ready remove and serve

NOODLE SOUP

Serves: 2

Prep Time: **10** Minutes

Cook Time: **40** Minutes

Total Time: **50** Minutes

INGREDIENTS

- 1L vegetable stock
- 1 chicken breast
- 1 tsp root ginger
- 1 garlic clover
- 2 oz noodles
- 2 mushrooms
- 2 onions
- 2 tsp soy sauce
- Basil leaves

DIRECTIONS

1. In a pan add vegetable stock, chicken breast, ginger, garlic and bring to a boil, simmer for 20-30 minutes
2. When chicken is tender remove and shred with a fork
3. Return chicken to the pot, add noodles, mushrooms, onion, soy sauce and simmer until noodles are tender
4. When ready remove from heat and serve with basil leaves

POTATO SOUP

Serves: **4**
Prep Time: 5 Minutes

Cook Time: **25**   Minutes

Total Time: **30**   Minutes

INGREDIENTS

- 1 oz. butter
- 3-4 rashers bacon
- 1 onion
- 1 lb. leek
- 2 potatoes
- 1L vegetable stock
- ¼ lb. cream

DIRECTIONS

1. In a pan fry bacon and onion in melted butter until golden brown
2. Add leeks, potatoes and cook for 5-6 minutes
3. Pour in the stock, bring to a boil and simmer until vegetables are soft
4. When ready remove, blend until smooth and serve with bacon

BOLOGNESE SOUP WITH PENNE

Serves: **4**

Prep Time: **5** Minutes

Cook Time: **40** Minutes

Total Time: **45** Minutes

INGREDIENTS

- 2 tsp olive oil
- 2 onions
- 2 carrots
- 2 celery sticks
- 2 garlic cloves
- 1 pack steak mince
- 1 lb. carton passata
- 1 tablespoon bouillon powder
- 1 tsp paprika
- ¼ lb. penne
- 1 oz. parmesan cheese

DIRECTIONS

1. In a pan add onions, celery, garlic, carrots and fry until soft
2. Add the meat, passata, bouillon, 1L water, thyme, paprika and simmer for 20 minutes
3. Tip in the penne and cook for another 15-18 minutes
4. When ready remove from heat and serve with parmesan cheese

CORIANDER SOUP

Serves: *4*
Prep Time: *10* Minutes
Cook Time: *30* Minutes
Total Time: *40* Minutes

INGREDIENTS

- 1 tablespoon vegetable oil
- 1 onion
- 1 tsp coriander
- 1 potato
- 1 lb. carrots
- 1L vegetable stock
- Handful coriander

DIRECTIONS

1. In a pan add onion, coriander, potato, carrots, chicken stock and bring to a boil
2. Cover and cook for 15-20 minutes
3. When ready remove from heat and blend until smooth
4. Add salt and serve

PASTA SOUP

Serves: 2
Prep Time: 5 Minutes
Cook Time: 25 Minutes
Total Time: 30 Minutes

INGREDIENTS

- 1 tablespoon olive oil
- 1 carrot
- 1 onion
- 1L vegetable stock
- 1 lb. tomatoes
- ½ lb. beans
- ½ lb. peas
- 1 pack filled tortellini
- Handful of basil
- Parmesan cheese

DIRECTIONS

1. In a pan fry carrots and onion until soft
2. Add tomatoes, stock, beans, peas and simmer for 15-18 minutes
3. Stir in the pasta, basil and simmer for another 4-5 minutes or until pasta is cooked
4. When ready serve with parmesan cheese

CAULIFLOWER SOUP

Serves: **4**

Prep Time: **5** Minutes

Cook Time: **25** Minutes

Total Time: **30** Minutes

INGREDIENTS

- 1 tablespoon olive oil
- 1 onion
- 1 cauliflower
- 2 garlic cloves
- 0,7 L vegetable stock
- 3 tablespoons double cream
- 1 piece of chorizo

DIRECTIONS

1. In a saucepan add onion, cauliflower, ½ garlic and cook for 5-6 minutes
2. Add stock and cook for 10-15 minutes or until cauliflower is tender
3. In a frying pan fry chorizo, remaining garlic, and cook for 2-3 minutes
4. When ready blend the soup, add double cream and season with pepper

BROCCOLI SOUP

Serves: *4*
Prep Time: *10* Minutes
Cook Time: *25* Minutes
Total Time: *35* Minutes

INGREDIENTS

- 1 tablespoon oil
- 1 onion
- 2 sticks celery
- 1 leek
- 1 potato
- 1L vegetable stock
- 1 head broccoli
- 1 tablespoon butter
- ¼ lb. blue cheese

DIRECTIONS

1. In a saucepan add onion, celery stick, leek, potato, butter, cover with a lid and cook for 7-8 minutes
2. Add stock, broccoli and cook until vegetables are soft, 12-15 minutes
3. Add the rest of vegetables and cook until soft
4. When ready blend the soup until smooth
5. Stir in blue cheese and serve with pepper

CHEESE SOUP

Serves: **4**

Prep Time: **10** Minutes

Cook Time: **30** Minutes

Total Time: **40** Minutes

INGREDIENTS

- 1 tablespoon butter

- 1 onion
- 1 cauliflower
- 1 potato
- 1L vegetable stock
- 0,4L milk
- 1/3 lb. cheddar cheese

DIRECTIONS

1. In a saucepan add onion, cauliflower, milk, potato, stock and bring to a boil, simmer for 20-30 minutes
2. When ready blend soup until smooth
3. Top with cheddar cheese and serve

LENTIL SOUP

Serves: 4

Prep Time: 10 Minutes

Cook Time: 20 Minutes

Total Time: 30 Minutes

INGREDIENTS

- 2 tsp curry powder

- 2 tablespoons olive oil
- 1 onion
- 2 garlic cloves
- 1 pack coriander
- 1-piece root ginger
- 2 lb. sweet potatoes
- 1L vegetable stock
- ¼ lb. red lentils
- 0,4 L milk

DIRECTIONS

1. In a saucepan add olive oil, onions, garlic, coriander, ginger, stalks, and cook for 7-8 minutes
2. Add potatoes, stock, milk, lentils, and simmer for 20-25 minutes
3. When ready blend until smooth and serve with seasoning

WINTER SOUP

Serves: 3
Prep Time: 10 Minutes
Cook Time: 35 Minutes
Total Time: 45 Minutes

INGREDIENTS

- 1 tablespoon thyme leaves
- 1 leek
- 2 sticks celery
- 2 carrots

- 3 oz. red lentils
- 2 garlic cloves
- 1 tablespoon bouillon powder
- 1 tsp coriander

DIRECTIONS

1. In a pan add all vegetables and simmer over low heat for 25-30 minutes
2. Cook until vegetables are tender
3. Remo from heat, blend until smooth and serve with seasoning

ROASTED RED PEPPER & SWEET POTATO SOUP

Serves: 2
Prep Time: 10 Minutes
Cook Time: 35 Minutes
Total Time: 45 Minutes

INGREDIENTS

- 1 sweet potato
- 1 red pepper
- 1 onion
- 2 garlic cloves

- 1 tsp paprika
- 0,3 L almond milk
- 0,3 L vegetable broth
- ¼ tablespoon sriracha

DIRECTIONS

1. Place the sweet potato, onion, garlic, and pepper on a baking tray
2. Sprinkle with seasoning, paprika and toss together
3. Roast for 20-30 minutes at 375 F
4. Place the vegetables in a blender and blend until smooth
5. Add almond milk, stock, sriracha and blend again
6. When ready serve with seasoning

CELERY SOUP

Serves: **4**

Prep Time: **10** Minutes

Cook Time: **40** Minutes

Total Time: **50** Minutes

INGREDIENTS

- 1 tablespoon olive oil
- 1 lb. celery
- 1 garlic clove
- ½ lb. potatoes
- 0,4 L chicken stock
- ¼ lb. almond milk

DIRECTIONS

1. In a saucepan add garlic, celery, potatoes, water and cook for 15-18 minutes or until tender
2. Add stock, simmer for another 18-20 minutes
3. When ready blend until smooth, add milk and blend again
4. When ready serve with seasoning

TOMATO SOUP

Serves: 4

Prep Time: 5 Minutes

Cook Time: 35 Minutes

Total Time: 40 Minutes

INGREDIENTS

- 1 tablespoon olive oil
- 1 onion
- 1 carrot
- 1 celery stick
- 1 can tomatoes
- 0,4 L chicken stock
- ¼ lb. soup pasta

- Parmesan cheese
- 1 tablespoon cream

DIRECTIONS

1. In a saucepan add carrot, onion, celery and fry for 10-12 minutes
2. Add tomatoes, stock, water and simmer for 15-20 minutes
3. Stir in cream and cook for another 2-3 minutes
4. When ready remove from heat and serve with parmesan cheese

PIZZA

GRAIN-FREE PIZZA CRUST

Serves: **4**

Prep Time: **15** Minutes

Cook Time: **15** Minutes

Total Time: **30** Minutes

INGREDIENTS

- 2 eggs
- 2 tablespoons apple sauce
- ¼ cup coconut flour
- ½ cup almond flour
- ½ tsp salt
- ½ tsp dried basil

DIRECTIONS

6. In a food processor add the eggs and process until smooth
7. Add salt, coconut flour, applesauce, almond flour, and mix well
8. Mix until it forms a ball in the processor
9. Scrap the dough together into a ball, put the dough onto the parchment paper
10. Bake at 350 F for 15 minutes
11. Remove from oven and serve the pizza crust

ZUCCHINI CRUST

Serves: **4**

Prep Time: **10** Minutes

Cook Time: **10** Minutes

Total Time: **20** Minutes

INGREDIENTS

- 1 zucchini
- 1 egg
- ½ cup parmesan cheese
- ¼ cup coconut flour

DIRECTIONS

1. Preheat oven to 425 F
2. Grate zucchini, sprinkle with salt and toss well
3. Place the zucchini in a bowl with eggs, almond flour, parmesan cheese, salt and pepper
4. Pat zucchini mixture into a thin round and bake until golden brown (10-12 minutes)

BREAKFAST PIZZA

Serves: **4**

Prep Time: **10** Minutes

Cook Time: **15** Minutes

Total Time: **25** Minutes

INGREDIENTS

- 5 eggs
- 1 tablespoon lard
- 1 red capsicum
- 4 oz. ham
- ¼ cherry tomatoes
- ¼ cup black olives
- 1 handful of rocket leaves
- salt and pepper for seasoning

DIRECTIONS

1. Preheat the grill to 350 F
2. In a bowl mix eggs and season with salt and pepper
3. In a frying pan melt lard, add capsicum and cook
4. Add tomatoes, lard, ham, olive and stir for 1-2 minutes

5. Spread over the base of the frying pan
6. Pour in the egg mixture and reduce heat to low
7. Cook until the base has firmed
8. Remove from the grill and slice into wedges and serve

PIZZA WITH THE LOT

Serves: **4**

Prep Time: **10** Minutes

Cook Time: **20** Minutes

Total Time: **30** Minutes

INGREDIENTS

- 1 lb. ground beef
- 1 egg
- 1 tsp parsley
- 1 tsp dried basil
- ¼ tsp salt
- ½ tsp pepper
- ¼ cup tomato puree
- 1 tsp tomato paste
- ¼ red pepper
- 1 tsp dried basil
- ¼ cup olives
- 5 slices prosciutto
- 4 oz. parmesan
- 1 handful fresh basil

DIRECTIONS

1. Preheat the oven to 430 F
2. In a bowl add salt, mince, egg, basil, pepper, parsley and mix well
3. Roll into a ball and place on a baking tray
4. Bake for 12-15 minutes
5. Mix the tomato paste with tomato puree and spread across the base
6. Top with peppers, prosciutto, parmesan, olives and bake for another 8-10 minutes
7. Remove from the oven, top with basil leaves and serve

VEGGIE PIZZA WITH CAULIFLOWER CRUST

Serves: **4**

Prep Time: **10** Minutes

Cook Time: **20** Minutes

Total Time: **30** Minutes

INGREDIENTS

- Cauliflower crust
- 1 chicken breast
- 1 tablespoon garlic infused oil
- 1 carrot
- 1 cup cherry tomatoes
- 1 cup spinach
- 1 tsp rosemary
- 1 tablespoon basil
- ¼ tsp salt
- ½ tsp black pepper
- ½ tsp red chili flakes
- 1 cup parmesan cheese

DIRECTIONS

1. Prepare the cauliflower pizza crust
2. In a skillet add shredded chicken and cook for 4-5 minutes in garlic oil
3. Add carrot, spices, salt, tomatoes, spinach and cook for another 5-6 minutes
4. Remove skillet from heat, add basil and spread chicken mixture over cauliflower crust
5. Cover with parmesan cheese and bake for 10-12 minutes at 450F or until cheese has melted

CAULIFLOWER PIZZA CRUST

Serves: **4**

Prep Time: **10** Minutes

Cook Time: **20** Minutes

Total Time: **30** Minutes

INGREDIENTS

- 1 cauliflower head
- ½ cup coconut flour
- 1 tsp salt
- 1/5 cup parmesan cheese
- 2 egg whites
- ½ tsp Italian seasoning
- ½ tsp black pepper
- 1 tablespoon oil

DIRECTIONS

1. **Preheat the oven to 400 F**
2. **In a pot place cauliflower, water and boil until soft**
3. **Place cauliflower into a blender and blend**
4. **Scoop cauliflower into a mesh bag and squeeze excess water**

5. In a bowl mix all ingredients together
6. Spread cauliflower dough on a parchment paper
7. Place in the oven and bake for 15-20 minutes or until ready

COCONUT FLOUR PIZZA CRUST

Serves: **2**

Prep Time: **10** Minutes

Cook Time: **20** Minutes

Total Time: **30** Minutes

INGREDIENTS

- 3 eggs
- ½ cup coconut flour
- ½ cup milk yogurt
- 1 tsp onion powder
- 1 tsp dried oregano
- 1 tsp dried basil
- ½ cup parmesan cheese
- 2 cloves garlic
- ½ tsp sea salt

DIRECTIONS

1. Preheat the oven at 400 F
2. Whip the eggs in a bowl with the yogurt and salt
3. Add coconut flour and whip until smooth

4. Blend in the onion powder, basil, oregano, garlic, and parmesan cheese
5. Pour about ½ the batter onto a parchment paper and spread the batter
6. Bake for 10 minutes, remove from the oven and add pizza sauce and other toppings
7. Bake for another 6-8 minutes and repeat this process with remaining coconut batter

PIZZA ROLLS

Serves: **4**

Prep Time: **10** Minutes

Cook Time: **35** Minutes

Total Time: **45** Minutes

INGREDIENTS

- 1 cauliflower pizza dough
- 1 package of pepperoni
- 1 tablespoon crushed oregano

DIRECTIONS

1. **Preheat the oven to 375 F**
2. **Place the cauliflower pizza dough on a parchment paper and push the dough out to form a rectangle**
3. **Place baking sheet in the oven for 25-30 minutes**
4. **Remove from the oven and place a row of pepperoni and sprinkle with oregano on top**
5. **Cook for another 6-8 minutes**
6. **When ready, remove and serve**

ZUCCHINI PIZZA CRUST

Serves: **4**

Prep Time: **10** Minutes

Cook Time: **30** Minutes

Total Time: **40** Minutes

INGREDIENTS

- 4 zucchini
- 2 tsp salt
- 2 cups almond flour
- 2 tablespoons coconut flour
- 3 eggs
- 2 ½ cups parmesan cheese
- 1 tsp red pepper flakes
- 1 tsp dried oregano

DIRECTIONS

1. Shred the zucchini, sprinkle with salt and set aside
2. Preheat the oven to 400 F
3. Mix zucchini with remaining ingredients
4. Place the dough over a baking sheet and spread evenly

5. Pop the pizza crust in the oven for 30 minutes or until golden brown
6. When ready, remove and serve

SPAGHETTI SQUASH PIZZA CRUST

Serves: **4**

Prep Time: **10** Minutes

Cook Time: **30** Minutes

Total Time: **40** Minutes

INGREDIENTS

- 1 spaghetti squash
- 1 tablespoon olive oil
- 1 egg
- ¼ cup mozzarella cheese
- 1 tsp salt
- 1 tsp black pepper

DIRECTIONS

1. Preheat the oven to 375 F
2. Cut spaghetti squash in half and remove seeds, place on a baking sheet and roast until tender
3. In a bowl add squash, mozzarella cheese, parmesan cheese, egg, salt and black pepper
4. Press squash in a thin layer on a baking sheet
5. Bake for 15-20 minutes, remove from the oven

6. Flip, add toppings and cook for another 10 minutes
7. When ready, remove and serve

LOW CARB ALMOND FLOUR PIZZA CRUST

Serves: *4*

Prep Time: *10* Minutes

Cook Time: *30* Minutes

Total Time: *40* Minutes

INGREDIENTS

- 1 egg
- ¼ cup water
- 1 tablespoon olive oil
- 1 cup almond flour
- ¼ cup parmesan cheese
- ½ tablespoon baking powder

DIRECTIONS

1. Preheat the oven to 350 F
2. In a bowl mix all ingredients
3. Place mixture into a blender and blend until smooth
4. Roll up the dough to make a square and place onto a baking sheet
5. Bake for 20-25 minutes
6. When ready, remove and serve

SIDE DISHES

PAN SEARED SEA SCALLOPS

Serves: **4**

Prep Time: **5** Minutes

Cook Time: **5** Minutes

Total Time: **10** Minutes

INGREDIENTS

- 12 oz. sea scallops
- 1 tsp onion powder
- 1 tsp salt
- 1 tsp lemon juice

DIRECTIONS

1. In a pan place scallops and cook for 2-3 minutes each side
2. Squeeze lemon juice over scallops and continue to cook until done
3. When ready remove and serve

CHICKEN SAUTE

Serves: **6**
Prep Time: **10** Minutes
Cook Time: **20** Minutes
Total Time: **30** Minutes

INGREDIENTS

- 4 chicken breasts
- ¼ cup vegetable stock
- 1 clove garlic
- 1 cup almond milk
- 10 oz. spinach
- 1 heaping crimini mushroom
- 1 tablespoon onion powder
- 1 tsp salt

DIRECTIONS

1. Preheat a skillet over low heat
2. Add chicken breasts and cook for 4-5 minutes per side
3. Add stock, garlic, onion, onion powder, milk, spinach, mushrooms and bring to a boil

4. Add chicken back, reduce heat and simmer for 8-10 minutes
5. When ready remove and serve with parmesan

EGGS BENEDICT

Serves: 2

Prep Time: 5 Minutes

Cook Time: 15 Minutes

Total Time: 20 Minutes

INGREDIENTS

- 2 toaster waffle
- 1 triangle cow cheese
- 2 oz. chopped spinach
- 2 poached eggs

DIRECTIONS

1. Toast your waffles and spread cheese over
2. Top with poached eggs and spinach
3. Serve when ready

GINGERBREAD SWEET POTATOES

Serves: 2

Prep Time: 10 Minutes

Cook Time: 20 Minutes

Total Time: 30 Minutes

INGREDIENTS

- 4 sweet potatoes
- 1 tablespoon orange juice
- 1 tablespoon blackstrap molasses
- ¼ tsp ginger
- ¼ tsp cinnamon
- ¼ tsp nutmeg

DIRECTIONS

1. Grill your sweet potatoes
2. Mash sweet potatoes with the rest of ingredients and mix well
3. When ready serve with seasoning

HONEY ORANGE ROASTED BEETS

Serves: **4**

Prep Time: **10** Minutes

Cook Time: **40** Minutes

Total Time: **50** Minutes

INGREDIENTS

- 3 beets
- 2 tablespoons olive oil
- 1 tsp balsamic vinegar
- 1 tsp honey
- 1 tsp onion powder
- 1 tsp salt
- orange juice

DIRECTIONS

1. Preheat oven to 425 F
2. Roast beets for 40 minutes and set aside
3. Combine remaining ingredients to make the vinaigrette
4. When ready serve with roasted beets

POPTART CRUMBLE

Serves: 2

Prep Time: 5 Minutes

Cook Time: 45 Minutes

Total Time: 50 Minutes

INGREDIENTS

- 1 can sliced peaches
- 2 sugar cinnamon Poptars
- ½ tsp cinnamon
- ¼ tsp allspice

DIRECTIONS

1. Preheat oven to 375 F
2. In a baking dish add peach slices with orange juice
3. In a blender add Poptars, cinnamon, spices and blend until smooth
4. Cover peaches with Poptars mixture and bake for 30-40 minutes
5. When ready remove and serve

CRANBERRY GLAZED CHICKEN

Serves: **4**

Prep Time: **10** Minutes

Cook Time: **20** Minutes

Total Time: **30** Minutes

INGREDIENTS

- 4 chicken breasts
- ¼ tsp thyme
- 1 tsp onion powder
- 1 tsp salt
- 8 oz cranberry sauce
- ½ cup maple syrup
- 1 tsp balsamic vinegar

DIRECTIONS

1. Cut each chicken breast into two cutlets
2. Season cutlets with thyme, onion powder, and salt
3. In a saucepan add cranberry sauce and maple syrup over low heat

4. Grill chicken for 5-6 minutes per side, brush with glaze each side and serve the cooked chicken with remaining glaze

ROASTED CHICKEN BREAST

Serves: 4
Prep Time: 10 Minutes
Cook Time: 35 Minutes
Total Time: 45 Minutes

INGREDIENTS

- 2 chicken breasts
- 2 tsp onion powder
- 1 tsp salt

DIRECTIONS

1. Preheat oven to 400 F
2. Place breast on a sheet and season
3. Roast for 30-35 minutes
4. When ready remove and serve

KALE CHIPS

Serves: **6**

Prep Time: **10** Minutes

Cook Time: **25** Minutes

Total Time: **35** Minutes

INGREDIENTS

- 1 bunch of kale
- 1 tablespoon olive oil
- 1 tsp salt

DIRECTIONS

1. **Preheat the oven to 325 F**
2. **Chop the kale into chip size pieces**
3. **Put pieces into a bowl tops with olive oil and salt**
4. **Spread the leaves in a single layer onto a parchment paper**
5. **Bake for 20-25 minutes**
6. **When ready, remove and serve**

GARLIC HERB CRACKERS

Serves: **4**

Prep Time: **10** Minutes

Cook Time: **20** Minutes

Total Time: **30** Minutes

INGREDIENTS

- 1 cup almond flour
- ¼ tsp salt
- 1 tsp chopped herbs
- 1 tsp garlic oil
- 1 egg

DIRECTIONS

1. In a bowl mix almond flour, chopped herbs, and salt
2. Add wet ingredients into dry ingredients and mix well
3. Press the dough onto a parchment paper
4. Score the dough into 2-inch squares
5. Bake at 325 F for 12-15 minutes
6. When ready remove and serve

GASTROPARESIS COOKBOOK

40+ Breakfast, pancakes, muffins and cookies recipes designed for Gastroparesis diet

BREAKFAST

CHIA SEEDS WITH MAPLE SYRUP

Serves: *1*

Prep Time: *10* Minutes

Cook Time: *8* Hours

Total Time: *8* Hours

INGREDIENTS

- 2 tablespoons chia seeds
- 1 tablespoon oats
- 250 ml almond milk
- 2 pecan nuts
- 1 tsp maple syrup
- 2 oz. raspberries

DIRECTIONS

1. In a bowl combine all ingredients together
2. Leave in the fridge overnight
3. Serve in the morning

BAKED QUINOA WITH APPLES

Serves: 2

Prep Time: 5 Minutes

Cook Time: 10 Minutes

Total Time: 15 Minutes

INGREDIENTS

- 1 cup water
- ½ cup quinoa
- 1 egg
- 4 tablespoons applesauce
- ½ tsp cinnamon
- 1 tsp pecans
- ¼ cup apple
- 1 tsp honey

DIRECTIONS

1. In boiling water add quinoa and simmer for 10-12 minutes
2. In a bowl pour quinoa, add eggs, apple sauce, and cinnamon
3. Top with apple, honey, and pecans

FRIED HONEY BANANAS

Serves: 2

Prep Time: 5 Minutes

Cook Time: 5 Minutes

Total Time: 10 Minutes

INGREDIENTS

- 1 tablespoon coconut oil
- 1 banana
- 1 tablespoon honey
- 1 tsp cinnamon

DIRECTIONS

1. In a skillet heat oil, add banana slices and fry for 2-3 minutes per side
2. Whisk together honey
3. When ready remove from pan top with cinnamon and serve

PORTOBELLO EGGS

Serves: **4**

Prep Time: **5** Minutes

Cook Time: **30** Minutes

Total Time: **35** Minutes

INGREDIENTS

- 4 Portobello mushrooms
- ¼ tsp salt
- ¼ tsp black pepper
- ¼ tsp garlic powder
- 2 eggs
- 2 tablespoons parmesan cheese
- 2 tablespoons parsley

DIRECTIONS

1. Preheat broiler and set an oven rack in the middle of the oven
2. Spray the mushrooms caps with olive oil and sprinkle with seasoning
3. Broil for 5-10 minutes per side or until tender
4. When ready remove from the oven and switch to bake

5. Break an egg into each mushroom, sprinkle with cheese and bake for 15-18 minutes at 375 F
6. When ready remove and serve

GLUTEN-FREE BREAD

Serves: **8**

Prep Time: **10** Minutes

Cook Time: **3** Hours

Total Time: **3** Hours and 10 Minutes

INGREDIENTS

- ¼ lb. rice flour
- ¼ lb. buckwheat flour
- ¼ lb. gluten-free almond flour
- 1 tsp salt
- 2 oz. sunflower seeds
- 2 oz. pumpkin seeds
- 1 oz. sesame seeds
- 400 ml water

DIRECTIONS

1. In a bowl combine all ingredients together
2. Mix well using a wooden spoon and cover for 1-2 hours
3. Transfer the mixture to the loaf tin

4. Place the bread in the oven and cook at 400 F for 25-30 minutes
5. When ready remove and serve

BLUEBERRY JAM

Serves: 2
Prep Time: 5 Minutes
Cook Time: 15 Minutes
Total Time: 20 Minutes

INGREDIENTS

- 2 cups blueberries
- 2 tablespoons honey
- 2 tablespoons lemon juice
- 2 tablespoons chia seeds

DIRECTIONS

1. Coat blueberries with honey
2. Transfer blueberries to a pot and cook on low heat for 5-10 minutes
3. While cooking, add lemon juice, chia seeds and mix well
4. Cook for another 5-10 minutes and when ready transfer to jars

ALMOND SMOOTHIE

Serves: 1
Prep Time: 5 Minutes
Cook Time: 5 Minutes
Total Time: 10 Minutes

INGREDIENTS

- ½ cup almonds
- 1 cup apricot nectar
- ¼ cup apricots
- ¼ cup Greek yogurt
- 1 tablespoon almond butter
- 1 cup ice

DIRECTIONS

1. In a blender place all ingredients and blend until smooth
2. Pour the smoothie in a glass and serve

CLASSIC FRIES

Serves: 2

Prep Time: 10 Minutes

Cook Time: 30 Minutes

Total Time: 40 Minutes

INGREDIENTS

- 1 lb. potatoes
- 1 tsp salt
- 1 onion
- ¼ tablespoon coconut oil
- ¼ tsp chili powder
- ½ tsp salt

DIRECTIONS

1. Place potatoes in a saucepan and cover with water over low heat, boil potatoes until tender
2. In a skillet add coconut oil, toss onion and cook for 8-10 minutes
3. Transfer the onion to a bowl
4. Transfer the potato in a pot and cook for 2-3 minutes or until golden brown

5. When the potatoes are ready, add the onions, salt, paprika and the rest of the ingredients

CHERRY KEFIR SMOOTHIE

Serves: 2

Prep Time: 5 Minutes

Cook Time: 10 Minutes

Total Time: 15 Minutes

INGREDIENTS

- 2 cups milk kefir
- ¼ cup cherries
- 2 tablespoons honey
- ½ cup chocolate chips

DIRECTIONS

1. In a blender place all ingredients and blend until smooth
2. Pour the smoothie in a glass and serve

CAULIFLOWER TORTILLAS

Serves: **4-6**

Prep Time: *15* Minutes

Cook Time: *15* Minutes

Total Time: *30* Minutes

INGREDIENTS

- 2/3 head cauliflower
- 2 eggs
- ¼ cup cilantro
- ¼ lime
- salt

DIRECTIONS

1. Preheat the oven to 350 F
2. Cut cauliflower into small pieces and blend until smooth
3. Place the cauliflower in a microwave and microwave for 2-3 minutes
4. In a bowl whisk the eggs, add lime, cilantro, cauliflower, pepper and mix well
5. Shape 4-6 tortillas and bake for 10-12 minutes or until golden

BROILED GRAPEFRUIT

Serves: *1*

Prep Time: *10* Minutes

Cook Time: *10* Minutes

Total Time: *20* Minutes

INGREDIENTS

- 1 grapefruit
- ¼ cup honey
- 1-inch ginger
- banana slices

DIRECTIONS

1. Cut grapefruit in half and place them on a baking sheet
2. Drizzle grapefruit with honey
3. Place banana slices on top and coat with honey and dust with cinnamon
4. Broil for 6-8 minutes
5. When ready remove and serve

BREAKFAST QUESADILLA

Serves: **6**

Prep Time: **5** Minutes

Cook Time: **10** Minutes

Total Time: **15** Minutes

INGREDIENTS

- 1 peach
- 1 pear
- ¼ cup almond butter
- Pinch of cinnamon
- 1 tablespoon coconut oil
- 1 tablespoon raw honey
- 4 brown rice

DIRECTIONS

1. On a tortilla spread almond butter and top with pears and peaches
2. Drizzle with honey and place another tortilla over it
3. In a skillet place "tortilla quesadilla" in melted butter and cook until golden brown
4. When ready remove, dust cinnamon and serve

BAKED PEARS WITH WALNUTS

Serves: 2
Prep Time: 5 Minutes
Cook Time: 30 Minutes
Total Time: 35 Minutes

INGREDIENTS

- 2 pears
- ¼ tsp cinnamon
- 1 tsp honey
- ½ cup walnuts

DIRECTIONS

1. Cut pears and place on a baking sheet
2. Sprinkle with cinnamon, top with walnuts and cinnamon
3. Bake for 25-30 minutes
4. When ready remove and serve

MOZZARELLA AND EGG BAKE

Serves: 4

Prep Time: 15 Minutes

Cook Time: 35 Minutes

Total Time: 50 Minutes

INGREDIENTS

- 4 oz. baby kale
- 1 tsp olive oil
- 1 cup grated mozzarella cheese
- ¼ cup green onion
- 4 eggs
- 1 tsp seasoning
- Salt

DIRECTIONS

1. In a frying pan add kale and cook for 2-3 minutes
2. Transfer to a casserole dish, layer the grated cheese and add onions
3. In a bowl combine eggs with seasoning and pour egg mixture over the kale and stir well
4. Bake for 30-35 minutes at 350 F

MORNING CARROT MILKSHAKE

Serves: **1**

Prep Time: **5** Minutes

Cook Time: **5** Minutes

Total Time: **10** Minutes

INGREDIENTS

- 1 cup carrots
- 1 cup coconut milk
- 1 cup protein powder
- 1-inch turmeric
- 1-inch ginger
- ¼ tsp cinnamon

DIRECTIONS

1. In a blender place all ingredients and blend until smooth
2. Pour the smoothie in a glass and serve

BREAKFAST PEPPERS

Serves: 2
Prep Time: 15 Minutes
Cook Time: 25 Minutes
Total Time: 40 Minutes

INGREDIENTS

- 1 red bell pepper
- 2 strips turkey bacon
- 1 tablespoon onion
- ¼ tsp garlic
- 1 tablespoon tomato
- ¼ cup spinach
- ¼ tsp pepper
- 2 eggs
- 2 egg whites
- 1 tablespoon milk

DIRECTIONS

1. Cut the pepper in half lengthwise
2. Place the peppers on a baking sheet and roast for 10 minutes or until soft at 400 F

3. In a pan cook the bacon until crispy, reduce the heat and add onion, garlic, spinach and tomato
4. Cook until spinach is soft
5. In a bowl combine milk, egg whites, eggs, cooked bacon, vegetables, cheese and mix together
6. Pour egg mixture into the peppers and bake for another 20-30 minutes
7. When ready remove and serve

AVOCADO BACON AND EGGS

Serves: 2
Prep Time: 5 Minutes
Cook Time: 20 Minutes
Total Time: 25 Minutes

INGREDIENTS

- 2 eggs
- 1 avocado
- 1-piece bacon
- 1 tablespoon low-fat cheese
- Salt

DIRECTIONS

1. Cut avocado in half, scoop out some of the avocado
2. Crack an egg and pour inside of your avocado
3. Sprinkle with cheese, bacon, and salt
4. Cook for 15-18 minutes at 400 F
5. When ready remove and serve

APRICOT PROTEIN BAR

Serves: **6**

Prep Time: **15** Minutes

Cook Time: **25** Minutes

Total Time: **40** Minutes

INGREDIENTS

- ¼ lb. apricot
- 2 oz. oats
- 2 oz. desiccated coconut
- 1 oz. sunflower seed
- 1 tablespoon sesame seeds
- 1 oz. cranberries
- 2 tablespoons protein powder

DIRECTIONS

1. In a blender add apricots and blend until smooth
2. Add water, oats and blend again
3. Toast coconut, sesame and sunflower seeds
4. Stir seeds and coconut into the apricots, add cranberries, chia seeds, hemp powder and mix well
5. Roll into a bar and refrigerate before serving

OAT PORRIDGE

Serves: 1
Prep Time: 5 Minutes
Cook Time: 15 Minutes
Total Time: 20 Minutes

INGREDIENTS

- 1 oz. oats
- 200 ml coconut milk
- 2 tsp sunflower seeds
- 1 tsp vanilla sugar

DIRECTIONS

1. In a saucepan add oats, water and bring to a boil
2. Reduce heat and simmer for 5-10 minutes
3. In a pan add sunflower seeds and roast for 4-5 minutes
4. Stir in oats mixture roasted sunflower seeds, milk, sugar and mix well
5. Top with fruits and serve

COOKIES

BUTTER COOKIES

Serves: **12**

Prep Time: **5** Minutes

Cook Time: **15** Minutes

Total Time: **20** Minutes

INGREDIENTS

- 2 cups almond flour
- ¼ tsp salt
- ¼ tsp baking soda
- ¼ tsp butter
- 4 tablespoons honey
- 2 tsp vanilla extract

DIRECTIONS

1. Preheat the oven to 325 F
2. In a bowl combine dry ingredients with wet ingredients and mix until fully incorporated
3. Set aside for 50-60 minutes
4. Roll into small balls and press them on a cookie sheet

5. Bake for 10-12 minutes or until golden brown
6. When ready, remove and serve

PANCAKES

ALMOND PANCAKES

Serves: **4**

Prep Time: **5** Minutes

Cook Time: **15** Minutes

Total Time: **20** Minutes

INGREDIENTS

- 1 cup almond flour
- ¼ cup rice flour
- ¼ cup sugar
- ¼ tsp salt
- 1 tsp baking powder
- 2 eggs
- 1 cup almond milk
- 1 tsp lemon zest
- ¼ cup almonds

DIRECTIONS

1. In a bowl combine all ingredients together and whisk to combine

4. Spoon ¼ batter and cook for 2-3 minutes per side
5. When ready remove and serve

OATMEAL PANCAKES

Serves: **4**

Prep Time: **5** Minutes

Cook Time: **15** Minutes

Total Time: **20** Minutes

INGREDIENTS

- 1 tablespoon flaxseed meal
- 2 tablespoons water
- ¼ cup rice flour
- ¼ cup oats
- 1 tablespoon agave nectar
- 1 tsp baking powder
- ¼ tsp baking soda
- ¼ tsp salt
- 1 tsp lemon juice
- ¼ cup almond milk
- Maple syrup
- 1 cup blueberries

DIRECTIONS

1. In a blender add oats and blend until smooth
2. In another bowl combine all ingredients together with blended oats
3. Pour ¼ cup batter in a heated skillet and cook for 2-3 minutes per side
4. When ready remove and serve

CLASSIC PANCAKES

Serves: **4**

Prep Time: **5** Minutes

Cook Time: **15** Minutes

Total Time: **20** Minutes

INGREDIENTS

- 2 cups all-purpose flour
- 1 tsp baking powder
- ½ tsp salt
- 1 tsp sugar
- 2 eggs
- 1 cup milk
- 1 tablespoon butter

DIRECTIONS

1. In a bowl combine all ingredients together
2. Mix until there are no lumps
3. In a skillet melt butter and pour ¼ cup batter
4. Cook each pancake for 2-3 minutes per side
5. When ready remove and serve

FLUFFY PANCAKES

Serves: *4*
Prep Time: *10* Minutes
Cook Time: *15* Minutes
Total Time: *25* Minutes

INGREDIENTS

- ¼ cup milk
- 1 tablespoon white vinegar
- 1 cup flour
- 1 tablespoon brown sugar
- 1 tsp baking powder
- ¼ tsp baking soda
- 2 eggs
- 1 tablespoon butter

DIRECTIONS

1. In a bowl combine all ingredients together
2. In a skillet melt butter and pour ¼ cup batter
3. Cook each pancake for 2-3 minutes per side
4. When ready remove and serve

BUTTERMILK PANCAKES

Serves: **4**

Prep Time: **10** Minutes

Cook Time: **10** Minutes

Total Time: **20** Minutes

INGREDIENTS

- 1 cup flour
- 1 tsp salt
- 1 tsp baking soda
- 1 egg
- 1 cup buttermilk
- 1 tablespoon butter

DIRECTIONS

1. Preheat a skillet
2. In a bowl combine baking soda, salt, flour and mix well
3. Add buttermilk, butter, egg and combine well
4. Melt butter in a skillet and pour ¼ cup batter
5. Cook for 1-2 minutes per side
6. When ready remove and serve

RASPBERRY PANCAKES

Serves: 4
Prep Time: 5 Minutes
Cook Time: 15 Minutes
Total Time: 20 Minutes

INGREDIENTS

- ¼ lb. plain flour
- 2 eggs
- 300 ml milk
- 1 tablespoon coconut oil
- 1 tsp brown sugar
- 1 cup raspberries
- maple syrup

DIRECTIONS

1. In a bowl combine all ingredients together
2. Fold in raspberries
3. In a skillet melt butter and pour ¼ cup batter
4. Cook for 2-3 minutes per side
5. When ready remove and serve with maple syrup

BERRY PANCAKES

Serves: **4**

Prep Time: **10** Minutes

Cook Time: **10** Minutes

Total Time: **20** Minutes

INGREDIENTS

- 1 cup all-purpose flour
- 1 tablespoon brown sugar
- 1 tsp baking powder
- 1 tsp baking soda
- 1 cup milk
- 2 eggs
- 1 tablespoon butter
- 1 cup berries

DIRECTIONS

1. In a bowl combine all ingredients together
2. Fold in berries
3. In a skillet melt butter and pour ¼ cup batter
4. Cook for 1-2 minutes per side
5. When ready remove and serve

BANANA PANCAKES

Serves: **4**

Prep Time: **5** Minutes

Cook Time: **15** Minutes

Total Time: **20** Minutes

INGREDIENTS

- 1 cup flour
- 1 tsp sugar
- 1 tsp baking powder
- 1 egg
- 1 banana
- ¼ cup milk
- 1 tsp butter

DIRECTIONS

1. In a bowl combine all ingredients together
2. Mash banana and combine with the rest of the ingredients
3. In a skillet melt butter and pour ¼ cup batter
4. Cook for 1-2 minutes per side
5. When ready remove and serve

VEGAN PANCAKES

Serves: **4**

Prep Time: **5** Minutes

Cook Time: **10** Minutes

Total Time: **15** Minutes

INGREDIENTS

- 1 cup all-purpose flour
- 1 tablespoon brown sugar
- 1 tsp baking powder
- ¼ tsp salt
- 1 cup water
- 1 tablespoon oil

DIRECTIONS

1. In a bowl combine baking powder, salt, sugar, flour and combine well
2. Whisk the water and mix well
3. In a skillet heat oil and cook each pancake for 1-2 minutes per side

OATMEAL-BANANA PANCAKES

Serves: **4**
Prep Time: **5** Minutes
Cook Time: **15** Minutes
Total Time: **20** Minutes

INGREDIENTS

- 1 cup oatmeal
- ¼ cup almond milk
- ½ cup almond flour
- 1 banana
- 1 tablespoon brown sugar
- 1 tsp vanilla extract
- Pinch of cinnamon
- ¼ tsp baking powder

DIRECTIONS

1. In a blender place oats and blend until smooth
2. Mash a banana and combine with the rest of the ingredients
3. In a skillet pour ¼ cup batter and cook for 1-2 minutes per side

MUFFINS

PUMPKIN PIE MUFFINS

Serves: **6**

Prep Time: **10** Minutes

Cook Time: **20** Minutes

Total Time: **30** Minutes

INGREDIENTS

- ¼ almond butter
- ¼ cup canned pumpkin
- 1 egg
- 4 tablespoons honey
- ¼ cup oats
- 1 tablespoon flaxseed
- 1 tsp cinnamon
- ¼ tsp nutmeg
- ¼ tsp cloves
- ¼ tsp baking soda
- ½ cup chocolate chips

DIRECTIONS

1. In a bowl combine, all ingredients except chocolate chips
2. Blend the mixture until smooth and then fold in chocolate chips
3. Distribute the batter evenly among each muffin cup, fill each one about ¾
4. Bake for 15-20 minutes
5. When ready remove and serve

5 MINUTE MUFFINS

Serves: **4**

Prep Time: **5** Minutes

Cook Time: **5** Minutes

Total Time: **10** Minutes

INGREDIENTS

- 1 cup butter
- 2 bananas
- 2 eggs
- 1 tsp vanilla
- 8 drops stevia
- ¼ tsp baking soda
- 1 tsp apple cider vinegar

DIRECTIONS

1. Place all ingredients in a blender and blend until smooth
2. Pour batter into muffin tins
3. Bake for 5-10 minutes at 400 F
4. When ready remove and serve

BANANA MUFFINS

Serves: *12*

Prep Time: *10* Minutes

Cook Time: *30* Minutes

Total Time: *40* Minutes

INGREDIENTS

- 1 cup almond flour
- 1 cup pecan pieces
- 1 tsp cinnamon
- ¼ tsp nutmeg
- ¼ tsp baking powder
- ½ tsp salt
- 2 bananas
- 1 tablespoon honey
- 2 eggs

DIRECTIONS

1. Preheat the oven to 400 F
2. In a food processor add pecan pieces, cinnamon, almond flour, nutmeg, baking powder, salt and process for 45-60 seconds

3. Mush bananas, add honey, eggs and mix well
4. Add the flour mixture to the egg mixture and mix well
5. Scoop the batter into 12 muffin cups
6. Bake for 22-25 minutes or until ready

EGG MUFFINS

Serves: *8*

Prep Time: *10* Minutes

Cook Time: *60* Minutes

Total Time: *70* Minutes

INGREDIENTS

- ¼ tsp garlic powder
- 1 tsp salt
- ¼ cup hot sauce
- 4 eggs
- 1 green onion
- ¾ lb. chicken thigh skin

DIRECTIONS

1. On a baking pan add chicken thighs, season with salt and bake for 25-30 minutes at 400 F
2. In a bowl places the chicken thighs and shred, pour the sauce over and combine with the rest of the ingredients
3. Pour the mixture into muffin cups and bake for 25-30 minutes

4. When ready remove and serve

SIMPLE MUFFINS

Serves: **6-8**

Prep Time: **5** Minutes

Cook Time: **25** Minutes

Total Time: **30** Minutes

INGREDIENTS

- 1 cup flour
- 2 tsp baking powder
- 1 tsp sugar
- 1 egg
- 1 cup almond milk
- 1 tablespoon butter

DIRECTIONS

1. **Preheat oven to 425 F**
2. **In a bowl combine all ingredients together**
3. **Pour mixture in muffin cups and fill ¾ cups**
4. **Bake for 18-20 minutes or until golden**
5. **When ready remove and serve**

BLUEBERRY MUFFINS

Serves: **6-8**

Prep Time: **5** Minutes

Cook Time: **25** Minutes

Total Time: **30** Minutes

INGREDIENTS

- 1 cup flour
- 2 tsp baking powder
- 1 tsp sugar
- 1 egg
- 1 cup almond milk
- 1 tablespoon butter
- 1 cup blueberries

DIRECTIONS

1. **Preheat oven to 425 F**
2. **In a bowl combine all ingredients together**
3. **Fold in blueberries and mix well**
4. **Pour mixture in muffin cups and fill ¾ cups**
5. **Bake for 18-20 minutes or until golden**
6. **When ready remove and serve**

RASPBERRY MUFFINS

Serves: **6-8**

Prep Time: **5** Minutes

Cook Time: **25** Minutes

Total Time: **30** Minutes

INGREDIENTS

- 1 cup flour
- 2 tsp baking powder
- 1 tsp sugar
- 1 egg
- 1 cup almond milk
- 1 tablespoon butter
- 1 cup raspberries

DIRECTIONS

1. Preheat oven to 425 F
2. In a bowl combine all ingredients together
3. Fold in raspberries and mix well
4. Pour mixture in muffin cups and fill ¾ cups
5. Bake for 18-20 minutes or until golden
6. When ready remove and serve

ALMOND MUFFINS

Serves: **6-8**

Prep Time: **5** Minutes

Cook Time: **25** Minutes

Total Time: **30** Minutes

INGREDIENTS

- 1 cup flour
- 2 tsp baking powder
- 1 tsp sugar
- 1 egg
- 1 cup almond milk
- 1 tablespoon butter
- 1 cup almonds

DIRECTIONS

1. Preheat oven to 425 F
2. In a bowl combine all ingredients together
3. Fold in almonds and mix well
4. Pour mixture in muffin cups and fill ¾ cups
5. Bake for 18-20 minutes or until golden
6. When ready remove and serve

RAISIN MUFFINS

Serves: **6-8**

Prep Time: *5* Minutes

Cook Time: *25* Minutes

Total Time: *30* Minutes

INGREDIENTS

- 1 cup flour
- 2 tsp baking powder
- 1 tsp sugar
- 1 egg
- 1 cup almond milk
- 1 tablespoon butter
- 1 cup raisins

DIRECTIONS

1. Preheat oven to 425 F
2. In a bowl combine all ingredients together
3. Fold in raisins and mix well
4. Pour mixture in muffin cups and fill ¾ cups
5. Bake for 18-20 minutes or until golden
6. When ready remove and serve

BACON MUFFINS

Serves: **6-8**

Prep Time: **5** Minutes

Cook Time: **25** Minutes

Total Time: **30** Minutes

INGREDIENTS

- 1 cup flour
- 2 tsp baking powder
- 1 tsp sugar
- 1 egg
- 1 cup almond milk
- 1 tablespoon butter
- 1 cup bacon strips

DIRECTIONS

1. Preheat oven to 425 F
2. In a bowl combine all ingredients together
3. Fold in bacon strips and mix well
4. Pour mixture in muffin cups and fill ¾ cups
5. Bake for 18-20 minutes or until golden
6. When ready remove and serve

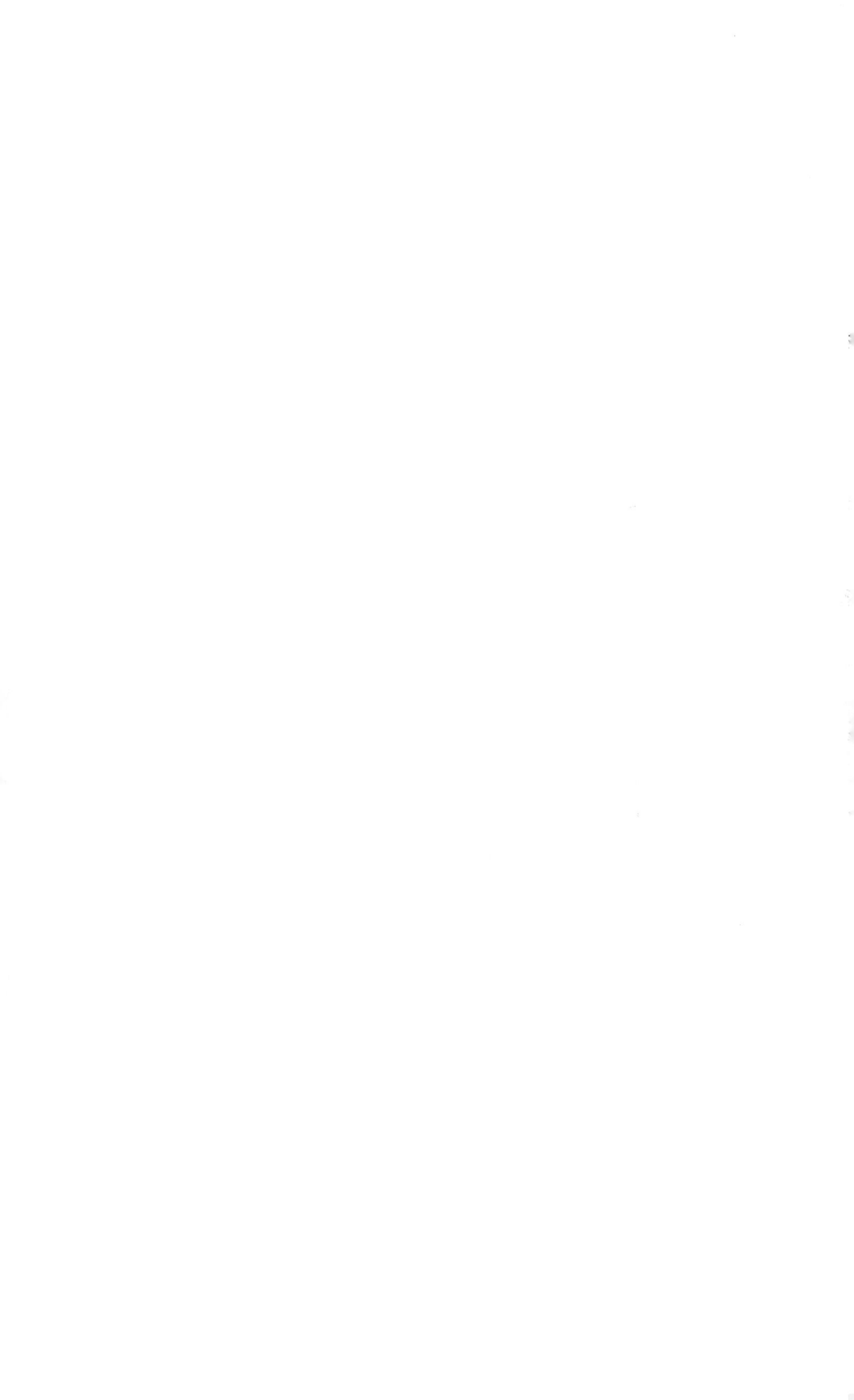

Made in the USA
Coppell, TX
06 December 2020